HERE'S WHAT PEOPLE ARE SAYI
DAVID CHOTKA, MAXIE DUNNAM,
AND *HEALING PRAYER*...

In one word: Wow! *Healing Prayer: God's Idea for Restoring Body, Mind, and Spirit* is not just about healing prayer; it breathes healing prayer! Through and through, this book is about the manifest presence of God in healing prayer. Worth the price of the book is the story in chapter 6 about a dying man who had accepted his fate and was planning his funeral, only to encounter God's healing presence manifested to him! Led by the Spirit, uniting two spirits as one, David Chotka and Maxie Dunnam do a masterful job of interweaving Scripture confirmed by signs, following and blending together Wesleyan and Christian and Missionary Alliance healing traditions. David and Maxie also write of God's comingling or intertwining of medicine and miracles (as well as beyond what medicine can do), what Oral Roberts called the praying hands—the hand of prayer and the hand of medicine as one. Dr. Chotka and Dr. Dunnam provide so many nuggets of practical biblical truth to describe features of healing prayer—such as "God initiates, we respond," "Embrace the mystery," "The intersection of human spirit and the Holy Spirit," and "The fiery manifest Presence of God"—and expressions of God's healing impartation: rising peace, forgiveness, compassion, love, touch, interior fire, prayer of tears—powerfully and practically illustrated through real-life encounters with the healing power of Jesus. This book covers the whole scope of healing prayer—physical healing—of the most difficult illnesses and injuries, healing from depression, trauma, fear, guilt, abandonment, bitterness, and more, as well as the "here now and not yet" of healing.

—*Paul L. King*, Th.D., D.Min.
Author, *God's Healing Arsenal*
and *Creating a Healing Community*

I stood in healing lines with Oral Roberts for six years. I experienced the healing power of the Holy Spirit on numerous occasions as I traveled the world. Yet there is a dearth of books written as primers for introducing healing prayer into the local church. Maxie Dunnam and David Chotka have given us a book written with compassion, faith, and hope. It is filled with testimonies, both biblical and contemporary, of the healing power of the Holy Spirit at work throughout the church. Read this book and be encouraged as your expectations are raised for teaching and experiencing the healing power of the Holy Spirit. Jesus is Lord, and the kingdom of God is afoot.

—*Dr. Robert G. Tuttle Jr.*
Professor emeritus, World Christianity
Asbury Theological Seminary

"What He did, we will do." That is the hope of this volume on prayer, from authors who have walked the walk. This book is full of stories that will encourage your faith and embolden your prayer life. Their definition of healing prayer as "an interactive, responsive relationship" will challenge you to move beyond words and formulas to an enlivened encounter with Jehovah Rapha, the God Who Heals You.

—*Rev. Dr. Carolyn Moore*
Founding pastor, Mosaic Church
Author, *Supernatural: Experiencing the Power of God's Kingdom*

This is a book that facilitates healing in groups. Easy reading, insightful, overwhelming, and excellent for the reader desperate to see that healing comes. The story of Elizabeth's healing is overwhelming and brought me to tears. Read it!

—*Rick Bonfim*
International speaker on prayer
Author, *Praying with Accuracy*

David Chotka and Maxie Dunnam provide a blend of theology, inspiration, and practical guidance to lead you into the ministry of *Healing Prayer*. If Jesus has risen, and Jesus is the same yesterday, today, and forever, then the true message is: This is who Jesus IS, and this is what Jesus DOES. *Healing Prayer* teaches and equips people to proclaim and practice that message!

—*Dr. Rob Reimer*
Director, Renewal Ministries International
Author, *Soul Care* and *Spiritual Authority*

This book is a practical and biblically grounded resource for ministers, prayer teams, and those who seek to bring healing grace to the whole person, whether physically, mentally, emotionally, or spiritually. Combining Scripture, reflection questions for those who minister, and their own life and personal experience, David and Maxie share how they wrestled with God and found keys to being God's instruments of change, healing, redemption, and reconciliation. This work challenges and encourages us to bless anyone, anywhere, any time.

—*Rev. Ken Graham*
President, Christian and Missionary Alliance of Australia

Accounts of healing from the hands of Jesus and the apostles, scriptural teaching on divine healing, testimonies from the healing ministries of the coauthors, instruction on how to pray for the sick and to train teams to carry it out, and finally practical wisdom on how to pray for the sick, including key dos and don'ts—*Healing Prayer* is a primer, a Healing 101, for everyone. Dunnam and Chotka show us how the supernatural can be quite natural in the life of the church. Healing the broken and the sick was a regular part of Jesus's ministry, as well as that of the disciples. Chotka and Dunnam believe that such a healing ministry should also be an ordinary part of our everyday ministry, among both clergy and laity. The coauthors bring their combined decades of experience in the pastorate to offer the reader down-to-earth, plain narrative accounts of healing that occurred not only in Christ's ministry but in their own. This book makes something like healing, which can seem complicated and intimidating, simple and accessible. The testimonies stir our faith as we are encouraged to walk in compassion as Christ did and reach out and touch the sick.

Healing Prayer seeks to impart faith and hope in the believer to pray for the sick and to build healing teams in the local church that will move in compassion and touch the broken, as the early church once did. The book is practical, offering wisdom from learned experience. It teaches believers how to prepare for healing ministry and identifies pitfalls to watch out for once they begin to pray for the sick. Dunnam, a Methodist, and Chotka, from the CMA tradition, like their spiritual fathers John Wesley and A. B. Simpson, are revivalists at heart. They recognize that the kingdom is demonstrated not only by word but also by deed and a demonstration of God's power to heal. The next revival in the West will need such a demonstration of the Spirit.

—*Dr. Peter J. Bellini*
Associate professor of evangelization
United Theological Seminary

David Chotka and Maxie Dunnam have joined together to craft a compelling and practical book on healing prayer. They approach the subject from the standpoint of both practitioners and prophets. They humbly articulate their personal challenges and uncertainties around divine healing. With powerful stories and startling supernatural encounters, they proclaim the undeniable truth that through God's empowering presence, we are invited to partner with the healing power of the Holy Spirit. This book creates anticipation and inspires imagination, boldly calling followers of Jesus Christ to be agents of God's healing touch to the nations.

—*Rev. Dr. David Hearn*
Past president, Christian and Missionary Alliance in Canada

For most of us, this book offers a completely new, inviting, and life-changing way to look at prayer. We are not trying to convince God; rather, we are sharing in His own heart and plan. The authors apply this paradigm to prayer for healing, showing us how we can pray with confidence that we are cooperating with God's plan and trusting that God hears us.

—*Dr. Craig S. Keener*
Professor of biblical studies
Asbury Theological Seminary

As we embrace increasing levels of brokenness in culture, the heart cry of many yearns for life-giving restoration of body, mind, and spirit. The relevancy of the book *Healing Prayer* is practical, applicable, and empowering for those who wish to serve as Christ's healing agents in an hour of chronic need.

—*Rev. Paul Lawler*
Senior pastor, Christ Church Memphis

HEALING PRAYER

GOD'S IDEA FOR RESTORING BODY, MIND, AND SPIRIT

DAVID CHOTKA and MAXIE DUNNAM

WHITAKER
HOUSE

HEALING PRAYER
God's Idea for Restoring Body, Mind, and Spirit

ISBN: 979-8-88769-062-9
eBook ISBN: 979-8-88769-063-6
Printed in the United States of America
© 2023 The Moore-West Center for Disciple Formation

Whitaker House
1030 Hunt Valley Circle
New Kensington, PA 15068
www.whitakerhouse.com

LC record available at https://lccn.loc.gov/2023029005
LC ebook record available at https://lccn.loc.gov/2023029006

CONTENTS

A NOTE TO THE READER

This manuscript has two authors. Both of us (David Chotka and Maxie Dunnam) agreed that we would use the term "we" to describe those moments when we are speaking of our shared theology and practices. We also agreed that any time one of us was giving testimony to our unique experiences and contributions, we would use the term "I" followed by one of our names in parentheses, Maxie or David.

We both affirm that our theology of healing is identical and that we are learning best practices from each other to pace each other toward a closer walk with Christ. In addition, we would like to express our heartfelt appreciation to Elizabeth Glass Turner for her significant contributions to this project.

Both of us completely agree that we owe a debt of gratitude for the dedicated work of two sets of people. Both teams labored tirelessly to bring this book to a broad constituency. Warm thanks belong to the Whitaker House team, namely Christine Whitaker, Amy Bartlett, Lois Puglisi, and our editor, Peg Fallon. Warm thanks also belong to the team at Journeywise for inviting us to expand a small startup idea into a larger, more complete work. Thank you, Shane Stanford and Nicolet Bell, for not only believing in this book but partnering with us to get it done. And we would be remiss if we didn't also thank Chip MacGregor for serving so diligently in his role to see this project brought to completion.

1

HOW WE DISCOVERED
"HEALING PRAYER IS GOD'S IDEA"

PART ONE: DAVID'S STORY

I had never met one. Not one!

Oh, I'd read about them in books and pamphlets; I'd heard about them in the media. I had even seen some strange-looking times of prayer for healing on television broadcasts of people who had called themselves "healing evangelists."

The problem was that I had just never met any.

After being a Christian for fully eight years, I had never personally met anyone who had experienced divine healing, whether that was physical, mental, or emotional healing sent from God and activated through prayer. In fact, I had never met anyone who had ever even prayed for another person to be made well with the expectation that God might bestow a supernatural gift of direct healing.

When I talked to friends about whether any "healed through healing prayer" people really existed, none of us were so sure. Many of my common-sense friends—the ones with *a good head on their shoulders*, the ones who understood something of life and thought clearly about how best to live—told me that such people probably didn't exist.

I wasn't so sure either. And therein lay the problem!

Not being sure of this put me in a conundrum because when I read about God's healing in Scripture, I was faced with the fact that those stories were there, especially in the life of Jesus of Nazareth. Naturally, when I read Scripture and reflected on a passage in which Christ would pray and someone would be healed, it gave me pause to consider whether some of those modern stories just might be true! After all, if they were included in biblical accounts, then whether or not I happened to see it personally, it became an *article of faith*, a matter of believing in the God who inspired the Bible.

The problem was deeper than that, however.

I knew about the forgiveness of God, and though I could not see it, I could see the effect it had on every kind of person. Those who were affected by God's forgiveness included the young and old, women and men, people of every race and nation, whether they were wealthy or middle class or poor. The ranks of the *forgiven forgivers* had among them not only the educated, but also those who scorned book learning, the intense, and the utterly indifferent.

Forgiveness from God and the command to practice it, which we could not see, became precious to them. This invisible forgiveness, being granted and practiced as a way of life, changed their lives, which *was* plain to see.

Do you understand the conundrum?

+ I knew about what I could not see—that God forgives us.

+ I knew it was true in believers of every kind—those who lived out the reality that God forgave them.

So there was evidence of the matter of faith that must be believed to be seen.

This brings us to the conundrum. Miraculous healing from God was recounted in the very same Bible that held the message of God's forgiveness. How then could I not consider that there should be evidence of God's healing now?

I wanted to meet someone, anyone, who had been healed or even had watched a healing occur, but those encounters eluded me. I lived *in the middle* between what I believed must be true and a complete lack of personal experience to that effect.

For eight years, I did not meet anyone who could testify to God's miraculous healing.[1] It was eight years, that is, until I wound up in the middle of a situation in which I myself was required to pray for someone. That one unexpected day turned out to be a game-changer, a paradigm-shifting moment that altered the course of the rest of my life.

To start the story, let me ask you a question: Have you ever prayed for someone to get well?

If you're like me, you may not have had a sweet clue about how to do it.

Not only did I not know how, but the first time I found myself asked to intercede for someone else's healing, it grated within me. This defining moment began with an emotional tug of war—I had no desire to pray for that at all!

Why?

The big reason was that I had never done it before, nor seen it done! That was a major consideration. Also, at the time, I didn't particularly want to be around the fellow who asked!

He later apologized...but this chap had regularly made fun of my faith, usually in front of peers who hung around him looking for a bit of humor to brighten their day. The fellow was a brilliant, insightful, and scathing jokester—and if you were the one on whom he aimed the scope of his humor gun, the trigger would be pulled, the salvo would be launched, a direct hit would be scored, and the room would explode with derisive, caustic laughter.

---

1. I did meet one young woman who had been at death's door after a car accident; she nearly died, with fifty-three bones broken in the collision and internal organ damage. Her neighbor happened upon the accident scene and was told by the medics on site that her heart had stopped. That neighbor, who had watched her grow up, found himself moved, so he suddenly prayed out loud for her heart to start beating—and suddenly, it did. However, emergency medics had already arrived and were administering CPR, so her survival could potentially be attributed to medicine alone.

At the time, I was a student in training for pastoral ministry. I believed the biblical accounts were true in every respect: Moses split the water, and Jesus walked on it. I believed then (and believe now) that these were physical, historical events.

The jokester didn't share these convictions; neither did most of our faculty members. So when I said, "The Bible is true; those events happened," the man would aim his scathing jester-bolt toward my verified location and, once I was firmly in his sights, he would fire off a volley that made the class (and invariably even me) laugh until it hurt.

And it usually did. Hurt that is. I was the object of his mockery.

In time, after too many of those moments, I just avoided him. So would you!

Then one day, I bumped into a mutual friend—a kind, gentle lady I'll call Susie. She told me the man was in the hospital. After a moment of expressing the hope that he would get well soon, she told me that the fellow had something to ask of me: He wanted me to come pray for his healing.

I was astonished, given our history. He had made fun of me just a few days prior for embracing this very thing. Not only was I flabbergasted, but I was more than a little afraid and immediately put up my guard.

I retorted, "No! I'm not going. I don't believe he wants me to pray at all." Vehemently, I added, "He just wants to mock again."

Susie paused and considered my words. After a moment, she agreed that he had been more than unkind, which was a frank admission from someone so considerate. She promised to confront him about his behavior and find out whether his request was genuine, and she left me at once so she could see him that very moment.

The next day, Susie bumped into me on our way to class. She shared that the man was truly sorry. He told her he felt badly about the way he had targeted me as an object of ridicule and was remorseful. The medical news had sobered him: he had a condition called phlebitis, and a blood clot was lodged in his vein. The result in 95 percent of the cases like this was that if the mass broke free, it would embed itself in the lung or brain. The outcome was always serious and usually fatal. It would kill him. He was young, in his mid-twenties, and wanted me to pray his life would be spared.

I had a kneejerk reaction—immediate, thoughtless, selfish, and completely unkind. I flat out told Susie, "I'm not going."

This evoked a response I had never seen before in calm, gentle Susie. To say she became *hopping mad* would be an extreme understatement. The usually mild-mannered Susie had fire in her eyes as she stomped her foot on the ground and vehemently said my name out loud, inserting my middle initial for emphasis:

"DAVID R. CHOTKA!"

I am sure my jaw dropped! Susie never talked that way to anyone! Her voice was raised, and her ire was profound. She nearly shouted the next part out loud.

"Do you believe that the Bible is the Word of God, or don't you? Aren't you telling everyone you meet that it is true and should be obeyed? How about this verse: *'I was sick, and you visited me?'*"

As soon as she said that, it was like a blow fell on the pit of my stomach. With a quiet interior moan, it became starkly, painfully clear that she was right; I would have to go, even if only out of sheer obedience to the Bible.

Later that day, as I entered his hospital room, it became plain the matter was more than serious. The space was packed with medical instruments; my jokester nemesis was hooked up to monitors, intravenous tubes, and wiring. He was pale, drawn, and obviously distressed. After a quick greeting, I asked him a simple question: "Why do you want me to pray with you when all you've done up to this point is make fun of the very thing you are asking me to do, to pray for healing?"

His voice was filled with anguish as he spoke haltingly, then in torrents. "I am so sorry I did that to you. Please forgive me! You need to know that you're the only person I know who believes the Bible is completely true."

I was stunned into silence.

Desperately, he added, "I have phlebitis, and I could die. I don't know anyone else who believes that God can heal. Won't you please pray for me?"

From this reading, you know that I had *never* done anything like that before.

- ✦ I had never seen it done!

- ✦ I had not one lone clue about how to begin!

- ✦ I didn't know anyone who had been healed by God's divine intervention.

Yet the honest, heartfelt distress in the fellow's voice moved me to my depths. Suddenly, my heart overflowed with a desire to honor the Lord and to bless this man. I found myself actually *wanting* to pray.

However, I still had no idea how to begin. I did remember that Jesus placed His hands on people to ask God for their healing. With some hesitation, and after asking his permission, I placed my hand on this man's left arm over the afflicted spot and began to ask God to have mercy on him.

To this very day, I don't remember what I said. I am sure it was a jumbled, halting prayer because, after all, I had never done anything like this before. Still, it was an honest prayer, asking God to remove the clot from his arm.

It was like fiery compassion filled the air we were breathing. The very room filled with what I would later learn to call "the Manifest Presence."[2] It was as if we were inhaling heaven's mercy.

Then that fiery Presence filled my heart as my eyes brimmed over with hot tears of compassion. That burning fire coursed through my entire being and overflowed through my arm to enter his. He told me that his body filled with, "Presence...fiery, life-imparting Presence..."

---

2. Throughout this book, we use a capital P for the word *Presence* when it is clear it refers to the divine. It is our conviction that this makes it plain that the word refers to the Holy Spirit. The term "Manifest Presence" is a classic theological term. It refers to a tangible sense of God's power becoming evident to human senses. "Omnipresence" is the antonym, a classic theological term used to describe God's universal Presence everywhere, whether sensed or not. The sharp contrast between these two ways to understand God's Presence is found in Exodus 40. While constructing the tabernacle, the Israelites under Moses were being guided by the God they loved, though they neither felt nor saw God's Presence while they built the tent. As soon as all the elements were in place and consecration completed, the Presence became manifest. "*Then the cloud covered the tent of meeting, and **the glory of the Lord** filled the tabernacle. And Moses was not able to enter the tent of meeting because the cloud had settled on it, and **the glory of the Lord** filled the tabernacle*" (Exodus 40:34–35). A New Testament example of this is found in the healing ministry of Jesus. Here is one instance, just as the Lord was about to pray for someone's healing: "*One day He was teaching, and there were some Pharisees and teachers of the Law sitting there who had come from every village of Galilee and Judea, and from Jerusalem; and **the power of the Lord** was present for Him to perform healing*" (Luke 5:17).

He asked what I had done for that fire to fill his body.

I had no words.

What he didn't know was that *neither of us* had ever experienced anything like that before. I was so overwhelmed that I raced out of the room. I was terrified of two things: I was astonished at the divine Presence flowing into and through me, and strangely, I was anxious that he would mock me again.

> SUDDENLY, SOMETHING HAPPENED—AND BOTH OF
> US KNEW IT. THE CHANGE WAS TANGIBLE.

The very next day, late in the afternoon, he was out of the hospital room and back on campus. It was medically verified: the phlebitis had vanished, never to return. (Years later, he sent a note to me confirming this.)

I found out what had happened, just after I left in shock.

A nurse and I crossed paths. I ran out as she was going in to check on the patient. With fiery consolation flowing through him, he told her that Jesus had healed him. She told him there would need to be tests; since he was booked for them anyway, he said, "Let's go get them done."

They ran the diagnostics and to everyone's great surprise, his veins were completely ordinary. Not only was there no phlebitis, but there was no scar tissue, no signs of any form of affliction at all. He was well.

Back on campus, he told me of the astonishing results of those tests. Then he looked over his shoulders in both directions before saying, "That prayer changed my life."

What he didn't know was that it changed my life too.

You can't pray like that, then see and feel the effect, then examine the medical evidence before and after, and ever be the same. That moment made something clear, and it is reflected in our book title: *Healing Prayer: God's Idea for Restoring Body, Mind, and Spirit*. It certainly wasn't *my* idea!

And so was launched a journey of years to discover the ways God heals through believing prayer, how we should intercede, what we should avoid, and how we can live with those times when the answers don't seem to come to us, times when we surrender everything to what we call *holy mystery*.

That day, however, marked a significant beginning. It was the day when God invited both me and the healed student to join Jesus's school of ministry, beckoning us to share His compassion and learn how to practice praying for healing.

> FOR THE FIRST TIME IN MY LIFE, I HAD JOINED WITH JESUS'S COMPASSION FOR SOMEONE WHO WAS SICK AND FELT THE POWER OF GOD FLOW INTO ANOTHER TO MAKE HIM WELL.

PART TWO: MAXIE'S STORY

Our oldest grandson was married recently.

It was a joyful occasion for our family. Naturally, as he is a member of a pastor's family, the preparation and the wedding itself garnered its fair share of conversation. What thrilled me most was when I would mention his name, people would exclaim joyfully, "Nathan, that's the baby we prayed for!"

Nathan's story is a good one to couple with David's account of his first experience of healing prayer. The narrative he recounted is one of what we might call *instant healing*, and I believe in instant healing.

My story is of a longtime dynamic of healing prayer.

When Nathan was three months old, his parents (my daughter and son-in-law) noticed that his eyes were moving around a lot, never quite focusing on anything. They took him to a pediatric ophthalmologist, who told them that Nathan had a congenital problem called *nystagmus* and that his eyes would always basically be that way. He then dilated Nathan's eyes to conduct an internal eye exam. In a matter-of-fact manner, the ophthalmologist told Nathan's mother, Kim, that Nathan had another congenital problem called *optic nerve hypoplasia*. This is a very rare defect in which Nathan's optic nerves were only about half the size they needed to be for him to see normally.

"What does that mean?" Kim asked.

"Oh, well, of course," the doctor went on as if he were discussing the weather, "he'll never be able to see normally; it's an uncorrectable problem. He will probably have to go to a special school and things like that. But don't be too worried; sometimes it's only minor, and they can go to regular school and sit in front of the class and things like that."

Kim thought, *And things like that?! This is my son you are talking about!*

You can imagine the anguish of Nathan's parents, us grandparents, and those who knew and loved Nathan; it takes little thought to envision all the pain and frustration that followed.

When I got word of Nathan's illnesses, naturally I began to pray, and I invited other people to pray with us. The word went out on The Upper Room Prayer Ministry network, as well as the other networks of our family. People all over the nation began to pray for Nathan.

Still, despite our intercessions, after numerous tests, it was medically confirmed that Nathan in fact had both conditions: nystagmus and optic nerve hypoplasia.

At that point, there was nothing to do but to live with it and prepare for a little boy moving through life with very limited eyesight. To put this in proper perspective, you need to know that Nathan's father is a medical doctor. He and Kim understood the medical realities associated with this.

About a year later, they moved to Hartford, Connecticut, for a medical internship. They followed up with a doctor for Nathan there. He examined Nathan and was pleased with the outcome. Kim was reassured, but not overly excited. Then the doctor dilated Nathan's eyes.

"Great!" he said. "These optic nerves look nice and pink and healthy."

In a sermon Kim preached much later, she talked about this experience:

What? I thought. *Say that again!*

I almost dropped Nathan in astonishment. I suggested that maybe he should read the first doctor's report more closely; after all, he had used words like "thin" and "white" to describe the optic nerves. Well, the doctor was amazed because what he saw and what the first doctor reported were on opposite poles. And not only that, but the nystagmus that supposedly would never disappear had diminished remarkably. And now, while it is still there, it is not always very noticeable.

Of course, in the world of medicine, there must be confirmation as well as explanation. So we went to a third doctor to get his opinion, and he too agreed that there was no optic nerve hypoplasia. They were both baffled about the drastic difference.

When Nathan was first diagnosed, we told our friends and family, who in turn told their friends and families. Soon we were receiving letters from all over the world saying that Nathan was being included in the daily prayers of many, many people.

Kim concluded her sermon:

I realize that I'm treading on difficult ground here as I touch on the topic of the power of prayer. However, I'm reminded of today's lesson from the Hebrew Scriptures:

"'For My thoughts are not your thoughts, nor are your ways My ways,' declares the LORD" (Isaiah 55:8).

There is a divine mystery here that we cannot fathom in human terms. We cannot reduce God to a human scale, nor can we assume that because events such as this do not happen all the time that they don't happen.

As I have shared personally and publicly through the years, if anyone attempts to assess my contribution to the church and growth of our Christian walk, it will be found in *The Workbook of Living Prayer*, which grew out of my own deep need. *Abiding in Christ: the Way of Living Prayer* is a sequel to that book. Many of my books have grown out of my ongoing struggle and desire to pray effectively and live a prayerful life.

Though I believe I have contributed foundationally to people's commitment and growth in prayer, I had some reservation about partnering with David Chotka in writing this book. It is clear that throughout his time of service to Christ, he has received various manifestations of gifts of healing through prayer. But the recent reminder of Nathan's healing as a result of a community praying (and praying for a long time) caused me to change my mind.

THERE IS NO QUESTION: PRAYER AND HEALING ARE CONNECTED.

We both believe healing prayer is God's idea. God invites us all to embrace His invitation to intercede.

REFLECT AND RECORD

1. What has your experience in prayer for healing been like? Does your church or fellowship group practice it?

_____

_____

_____

2. In the first account, David didn't want to pray for the man's healing. He went anyway out of obedience to Christ. What does this tell us about willingness to follow the Holy Spirit?

_____

_____

_____

3. Both the pray-er and the recipient of prayer felt something neither had felt before. It was a combination of compassion, fiery Presence,

and a sense of being commanded, all at once. Have you ever felt God's healing power flow? What was your experience?

_____

_____

_____

4. When you think of willingness to share God's compassion and to show up, how might this testimony encourage the daily practice of your faith?

_____

_____

_____

5. In Maxie's example, many people prayed, often from a great distance away. Many of them had never even met Nathan. There was no clearly distinct *healing anointing* or *instant knowing* that was a part of David's story. Yet, in time, a medically impossible healing occurred, to everyone's great joy! What does this tell us about healing prayer?

_____

_____

_____

A PRAYER TO BE WILLING

Lord Jesus, the Gospels give many examples of healing power flowing through You. Let me be open to Your compassionate power in and through me, whether I sense a healing anointing when I am before someone ill, whether I am unsure of how to pray, or whether I am praying from a distance. I give You myself; use my heart, hands, and voice to pray in whatever way You choose. Amen.

2

OUR CHURCHES AND HEALING PRAYER

This book is about something near and dear to our hearts: it is about sick people getting well, something all of us yearn to see. It is a focus on the prayer life of the contemporary church and an examination of the prayer life of Jesus of Nazareth, especially His ministry of prayer for healing. It is about how Jesus's ministry of physical, mental, and emotional restoration continues through ordinary people like you and me. In fact, this book is about how praying for healing should be a common practice for every believer in every branch of the Lord's church. Sadly, in many sections of the Lord's church across the earth, it's not.

As Rev. Carolyn Moore writes in the introduction to *Supernatural: Experiencing the Power of God's Kingdom*:

> I am hungry to see the power of the Holy Spirit in our midst. I'm not talking about so much that passes these days for Spirit-filled experiences. We talk of huge moves of God that are not quantified by fruit, and we call our good feelings "moves of the Spirit." We sometimes misrepresent the Spirit by assigning to him feats easily accomplished in the natural. Meanwhile, we are completely short-changing what must surely be a much more awesome and beautiful power than fleeting experiences. What is most disturbing is that we cling to stories of Holy Spirit power in other places at other

times, as if by having only heard the stories we can somehow claim participation. I am hungry for the power of the Holy Spirit to fall on us...here.[3]

In the early years of our respective walks with God, we (Maxie and David) did not see divine healing. Many churches didn't even attempt to pray for supernatural healing of the sick—at least they didn't pray with an expectation that God might transcend ordinary, natural processes by making someone well through believing intercession.

Was there compassion for the ill, wounded, pain-racked, and helpless, though? The answer is a hands-down, slam dunk *yes!* Most certainly!

Many good-hearted congregations displayed genuine yearning for sick people to become well. In our ministerial experience, this was reflected in magnificent acts of compassion, visitation, and ceaseless praying that God might see the injured or afflicted one through their time of trial. Our intercessions for them regularly demonstrated genuine longing that suffering people would be granted grace to endure. We would pray enduring grace for them until their body's natural healing powers (aided by medical science) would bring them to a place of health.

It is common today for congregations to entreat the Lord to bless medically trained specialists, doctors, nurses, and technicians to bring dearly loved sick ones to a place of health. And those prayers are good and valuable; they do not go to waste and should be continued.

Yet regularly in practice, it has become common for congregational prayers to be permeated with a phrase barely found in the New Testament. We have prayed it ourselves, and it's very likely that anyone reading this book will have prayed this prayer or some intercession similar to it:

"If it be Your will..."

I (David) have prayed that phrase when I didn't know what God's best was for the one I was praying about. I have also prayed it when I didn't know whether to ask God for healing, for a person to endure pain while natural healing processes, or for them to pass away because their time had come. It was an honest prayer. It sounds biblical. And I wanted to learn

---

3. Carolyn Moore, *Supernatural: Experiencing the Power of God's Kingdom* (Franklin, TN: Seedbed Publishing, 2020).

better how to pray. So I went into a study on the will of God, determining that I would sift through the biblical material on how to pray for the will to be done.

I DIDN'T FIND ONE CLEAR EXAMPLE IN THE NEW TESTAMENT OF ANYONE PRAYING "IF IT BE YOUR WILL." THERE WAS NOT ONE CLEAR CASE FROM MATTHEW TO REVELATION.

This phrase, "If it be Your will," is often associated with Jesus's prayer in the garden of Gethsemane. Yet there, Jesus knew exactly what God's will was; He bluntly told the disciples that He was going to die an awful death to save us. (See Mark 8:31–33; Matthew 16:21–23.) Moses and Elijah appeared to Him on the Mount of Transfiguration and talked to Him about just how He would die. (See Luke 9:28–36.) In fact, when Simon Peter understood what Christ was saying, he began to tell Him off. Jesus rebuked the well-intentioned fellow sternly and vehemently for telling Him that Messiah could not die like that! In fact, this rebuke was as strong as it ever got with Jesus speaking to another.

> *From that time Jesus began to point out to His disciples that it was necessary for Him to go to Jerusalem and to suffer many things from the elders, chief priests, and scribes, and to be killed, and to be raised up on the third day. And yet Peter took Him aside and began to rebuke Him, saying, "God forbid it, Lord! This shall never happen to You!" But He turned and said to Peter, "Get behind Me, Satan! You are a stumbling block to Me; for you are not setting your mind on God's purposes, but men's."* (Matthew 16:21–23)

It is clear from the Gospels that Jesus knew *exactly* what the will of God for His life (and death) was going to be. When He came to the garden of Gethsemane, Jesus was praying with a full and complete knowledge of what the will was going to be—and He foretold it in an exact, clear manner.

What was Jesus praying in Gethsemane?

With full and complete knowledge of the exact will of God for His life, He was asking for God the Father to create another way. Here is the logic:

- I know the will of My Father! I will be required to undergo a horrific, pain-filled death.

- Save humanity—yes I will, regardless of the cost!

- Yet is there any other way for this to happen? If so, send it!

That was the thrust of Jesus's prayer! Here is what we know about that holy prayer time just before the crucifixion:

1. Jesus knew the will of God.

2. Jesus didn't want the pain-filled pathway set before Him.

3. Jesus prayed for another way to save us.

4. God told Him, "No—there is no other way!" three separate times.

5. Jesus then embraced the will of God that had already been revealed to Him before that prayer time.

Jesus didn't pray, "If it be Your will," as we often do—as an escape clause in case there is no answer. Jesus prayed, "I know Your will! Can this be changed?" He prayed for the pathway to our salvation to be altered, fully aware that He would need to embrace whatever His Father would reveal to Him in real time:

> *"My Father, if it is possible, let this cup pass from Me; yet **not as I will, but as You will**…" He went away again a second time and prayed, saying, "My Father, if this cup cannot pass away unless I drink it, **Your will be done**." Again He came and found them sleeping, for their eyes were heavy. And He left them again, and went away and prayed a third time, saying the same thing once more.*
>
> (Matthew 26:39, 42–44)

Christ, fully human and fully divine, was wrestling with the prospect of what lay ahead. He was not praying from lack of knowledge as we often do in our intercessions.

Based upon Gethsemane, praying *"if it be Your will"* is *not* the same as praying, "I know what You are asking. Can this be altered? I will do exactly as You command."

On a different level, sometimes people who are praying the phrase "if it be your will" find biblical basis for the "if" from this passage found in 1 John:

> Now this is the confidence that we have in Him, that **if we ask any-thing according to His will**, He hears us. And if we know that He hears us, whatever we ask, we know that we have the petitions that we have asked of Him. (1 John 5:14–15 NKJV)

Yet this text is not an "escape clause" in case God doesn't answer our prayers as we hope; rather, this text conveys hope. It prods believers to pray with boldness based upon what they already know about the will of God. This is asserting before the Lord that a clear outcome (_____) *must* be done because they know that it is God's will!

THE ATTITUDE OF THE NEW TESTAMENT TOWARD PRAYING ABOUT THE WILL IS THAT WE ARE TO PRAY IN CONFIDENCE ABOUT WHAT WE KNOW THE WILL IS. AND WHEN WE DO NOT KNOW, WE ARE TO CANDIDLY ADMIT AS MUCH, THEN PRAY TOWARD KNOWING HOW GOD WOULD HAVE US PRAY.

There are no other texts in the New Testament in which we can find basis for an intercessor to pray, "God do this, if it be Your will."[4]

None.

---

4. It is possible to refer to Mark 1:40–41 in which a leper says to Christ, *"If You are willing, You can make me clean."* Yet Jesus Himself was the one who was doing the praying. He said, *"I am willing; be cleansed,"* and He placed His hands on him and prayed in confidence. The intercessor—in this case, our Lord—knew the will and prayed it.

It is far better to pray, "I am not clear on this. Guide my praying, Lord" than it is to pray prayers of uncertainty, such as, "Heal my friend, Lord, if it be Your will."

Churches are commanded to pray, for God has shaped the earth to respond to the prayers of God's people.

PRAYER THEN IS GOD'S IDEA.

This means God's people need to organize around training others to intercede. Many churches have developed approaches to train people to do just this. Both of us have done just that.[5]

Churches are also commanded to pray very specifically for the sick, the weak, the helpless, the afflicted, the emotionally distressed, the injured, and chronically ill.

HEALING PRAYER THEN IS GOD'S IDEA.

This means that churches need to organize training for people to learn how to intercede for the sick and the afflicted to bring healing to the whole person. This book is intended to do just that.

The Scriptures are filled with example after example of ordinary believers praying with the expectation that God will guide their prayers, even as they pray for those who need the touch of Christ to make them whole.

---

5. Maxie Dunnam's most important work is designed to train others to intercede. See Maxie Dunnam, *The Workbook of Living Prayer* (Nashville, TN: Upper Room, 1994). David Chotka's first book was designed to mirror the structure of Maxie's book and examines the teaching of each key word of the Lord's Prayer. See David Chotka, *Power Praying* (Terre Haute, IN: PrayerShop, 2009). David's work has been used as the primary anchor text for the *Transform Prayer Course*, available at www.alliancepray.ca in English, French, Mandarin, and Cantonese.

It is no exaggeration to indicate that those who love God and the Scriptures long for the power of the same Holy Spirit who was granted to Jesus of Nazareth. In fact, a very strong case can be made that the principal reason Jesus came was to fill us with Himself! Paul says it magnificently in Colossians.

For in Him dwells all the fullness of the Godhead bodily; and you are complete in Him. (Colossians 2:9–10 NKJV)

Wow!

Jesus came to send His very essence, His being, His very Spirit to fill us up with all the fullness of God—to make us complete. Now that's a destiny to live for!

ALL OF GOD WAS IN ALL OF JESUS. AND ALL OF GOD IN HIM GETS TRANSFERRED TO ALL OF US! HE MAKES US COMPLETE WHEN WE ARE "ALL IN HIM."

God's Spirit was poured out on throngs of early believers who, with magnificent expectation, followed the Lord in the early church and the generations that followed. The first generations of believers came to faith as the gospel expanded from those gathered in prayer at Pentecost to all points of the inhabited world, and they brought healing prayer with them.

The Holy Spirit moved in power through their witness to Jesus's resurrection. The book of Acts overflows with accounts of focused prayer, signs, wonders, and miraculous healings. It was ordinary to trust Christ in praying about everything! That includes seeking God for a clear word about how we should pray for His will to be done.

When the two of us met, we became prayer partners and friends. In time, Maxie spoke in churches that David had served. There, the two of us discussed our parallel projects on this topic: David had developed a short guide to train his altar prayer team in prayer for healing, and Maxie had developed a worship service of "praise, healing prayer, and Holy

Communion" for use in intercessory prayer. We combined our resources and merged them into a pamphlet. In time, we expanded that pamphlet and added testimonies from our ministries and churches. The result of that shared emphasis is this book.

Some of the practices we describe were forged in the school of hard knocks, as in David's story in chapter 1 in which someone who was desperately ill unexpectedly asked for prayer for healing.

Some of the convictions driving this resource were fueled when Maxie began to travel the world in ministry. He was stirred to discover throngs of believers across the earth who understood that healing prayer was to be ordinary. Maxie was moved by the revival of the gospel in places like Cuba, where prayer for healing is commonplace. In fact, revival regularly follows when signs and wonders take place as the gospel is preached.

It is our prayer that this book will be a resource, a tool to help you get started in praying with holy, humble compassion for people who are sick and afflicted, with the simple trust that we can rely on the words of Jesus with confidence: *"I came that they may have life and have it abundantly"* (John 10:10 ESV).

There is an important caveat to name as we journey together on this theme of prayer for healing.

THERE IS NO CONFLICT BETWEEN MEDICINE AND MIRACLE.

Over the course of our ministries, we have prayed and visited the sick in homes and hospitals. We have a high regard for the sacrificial gifts of scientists who have explored God's creation to unearth medicines and therapies to be used for the health and good of others. We are thankful for medicine, health care workers, and the labors of all those who care for the body and for mental health. We have also tasted something of God's power to heal supernaturally.

They did in the history of Judaism and in the ministry of Jesus. They also overlap and intertwine in the work of God's people everywhere.

> *MEDICINE AND MIRACLE OVERLAP AND INTERTWINE.*

This book is organized into user-friendly chapters, illustrated with testimonies of God's power to heal. Rooted in the Bible's clear testimony of God's power to heal, it is designed to offer practical insight on how to start praying with God's compassion for those who suffer.

Let's start the journey.

REFLECT AND RECORD

1. When you pray for people who are ill, do you usually pray for God to work through natural channels such as medical care? Do you ever pray for God to supernaturally intervene? Why or why not?

_____

_____

_____

2. Have you prayed for God to heal "if it be Your will?" Is there another way to pray for healing?

_____

_____

_____

3. Like Rev. Carolyn Moore, are you "hungry to see the power of the Holy Spirit in our midst"? What is holding you back?

_____

_____

_____

A PRAYER TO GROW IN TRUST

Lord Jesus, it is hard sometimes to follow You to places we do not understand. It may be easier to pray for doctors than it is to pray for Your immediate, intervening, mysterious act of healing. Thank You for the gift of medicine, for the gift of scientific inquiry into Your world, and for all who serve others and honor Your creation with their talents and work. But today, please show us that You still interact with compassion with the universe You created and sustain. Amen.

3

HEALING PRAYER—
SO WHAT DOES THE BIBLE SAY?

Churches across the world will do well to give the Acts of the Apostles a second look. In Acts, we discover the action of the Holy Spirit at work in the lives of believers. By receiving the Spirit of Jesus, they were empowered to carry out Jesus's ministry after the ascension. It is the account of the birth of the early church, which was released into the world through men and women saturated in prayer. Jesus promised this very thing:

You will receive power when the Holy Spirit has come upon you.

(Acts 1:8)

He told those fearful followers to wait in Jerusalem for the promise—and the promise was the reception of the third Person of the Trinity:

For John baptized with water, but you will be baptized with the Holy Spirit not many days from now. (Acts 1:5)

Those first believers suffered from no illusions about who they were! The memory of Judas's betrayal and even of their own abandonment of the Lord was very fresh. They knew the limits of their own power, and they did exactly as Jesus, the risen Lord, had told them to do. (Can you imagine having forty days of conversation with the Lord—after you watched Him die? It boggles the mind!)

That risen Lord told them to wait! So, they waited…

The actions of these early followers of Jesus, including His mother Mary and members of His family, are described in Acts 1:

All these with one accord were devoting themselves to prayer, together with the women and Mary the mother of Jesus, and his brothers.
(Acts 1:14 ESV)

You likely know what happened next:

Suddenly there came from heaven a sound like a mighty rushing wind, and it filled the entire house where they were sitting. (Acts 2:2 ESV)

We thrill at the way Luke the physician tells the story. He stumbles over himself as though he is grasping for words to describe what happened. And then, in a restrained way that seems to indicate that there was no ordinary way to describe what happened, Luke wrote it down. His words were crafted in a simple, straightforward fashion, in one of the most understated sentences in the whole Bible: *"And they were all filled with the Holy Spirit"* (Acts 2:4 ESV).

It was as matter-of-fact as that; they were all filled with the Holy Spirit.

Something astonishing and utterly new came into their experience. Out of those closed doors, these formerly timid, frightened men and women were transformed into bold proclaimers of the gospel. They started out in the very city that had crucified Jesus only weeks before. They went to tell of His resurrection and His life-imparting power to everyone they met.

To say that this is one of the most critical stories in the New Testament does not do justice to the history.

THERE WOULD BE NO CHRISTIAN CHURCH APART FROM THE MINISTRY OF THE HOLY SPIRIT WHO WAS POURED OUT AT PENTECOST.

The Holy Spirit continues to join our hearts and minds today to testify of all that has been done for us in Christ Jesus. And so, this brings us to the heart of the matter—and the centrality of the Spirit's Presence in our walk with God. To get at this, let us ask this question:

What is it that causes you to say, "I am a Christian"?

If we asked you that question in a personal conversation, you might respond by talking about what you believe. You might speak about your trusting in Jesus Christ as the foundation of being a Christian. There's a reason for this, of course; this is affirmed in Scripture.

The phrase, *"Believe in the Lord Jesus, and you will be saved"* (Acts 16:31) is quoted frequently by those who invite people into the Christian life. We say things like, "Believe in the Lord Jesus Christ" and "Accept Him as your personal Savior." Now there's basic truth in those messages. In fact, both of us personally responded to those texts, and it was meaningful for us.

But if it stops there, it stops.

To stop at that point is to shortchange the whole point of the New Testament.

That's where many Christians are stuck today. The gospel stops at the decision to receive the grace of forgiveness and *doesn't move us toward a divine infilling!* As a result, pews are full of people who believe in Jesus and affirm some kind of formal faith, yet those people remain empty and unfulfilled. They lack divine power while seeking (like John Wesley before his transformative Aldersgate experience) to obey God "under their own steam." For many, the transforming, empowering Presence of the Holy Spirit is not an ongoing part of their heart devotion, let alone their understanding and practice of the Christian life.

New Testament scholar Gordon Fee challenges us here. In his book *Paul, the Spirit, and the People of God*, Fee describes the preaching and power of the apostle Paul:

> The Spirit's role in Paul's preaching was not limited to an "anointing" of Paul's own words, thus carrying conviction as to the truth of the gospel.[6] In Romans 15:18–19 he insists that his preaching...

---

6. First Thessalonians 1:5 certainly joins preaching the gospel to an interior experience of God's power forming Christ within the new believer. Here is the NASB translation of the phrase: "*for our gospel did not come to you in word only, but also in power and in the Holy Spirit and with full conviction.*" Fee's point is that far more happened related to the activity of the Spirit when the message of Christ was preached by the apostle—and by implication, by us.

was an effective combination of "word and deed," both of which were by the "power of the Spirit."[7] By "word" he refers to his preaching; he explains "deed" as referring to the "signs and wonders through the power of the Spirit."[8]

Fee is making a bold claim.

He is stating that a major difference between the vigorous witness of the early church and the perceived irrelevance of the church today is due in large part to our current lack of a dynamic experience of the reality of the Spirit's Presence and power. There is a hunger, not for mere emotional experiences but for the very real Presence of God. So in offering this resource, part of our prayer is that people everywhere will pay attention to that hunger to receive *God's Empowering Presence*[9] by receiving the transformative power of the Holy Spirit.

We know that throughout the Gospels, healing prayer was regularly practiced by both the Lord and His disciples. (See, for example, Mark 6:12–13.) It often accompanied the teaching of Jesus; it was also imprinted in the life of the early church recorded in Acts. Healing is embedded in Paul's letters and the General Epistles, including his teaching on spiritual gifts. (The plural "gifts" is used when referring to healing in 1 Corinthians 12:9, 28, 30.)[10] Scripture beckons believers to the experienced infilling of the Holy Spirit's Presence and power; this includes gifts of healing from the Holy Spirit as a regular gift to the body of Christ.

---

7. *"For I will not presume to speak of anything except what Christ has accomplished through me, resulting in the obedience of the Gentiles by **word** and **deed**, in the power of signs and wonders, in the power of the Spirit; so that from Jerusalem and all around as far as Illyricum I have fully preached the gospel of Christ"* (Romans 15:18–19).

8. Gordon D. Fee, *Paul, the Spirit, and the People of God* (Grand Rapids, MI: Baker Academic, 1996), 78.

9. This is the title of the magisterial previous work by Fee on the Holy Spirit in the Pauline Epistles that led to the shaping of his shorter summary work on the Holy Spirit. See Gordon D. Fee, *God's Empowering Presence* (Peabody, MA: Hendrickson Publishers, 1994).

10. It is striking to notice that each spiritual gift named by the apostle in 1 Corinthians 12 is described in the singular, except this one. It is repeated three times in the plural. The best approach is that the gift is not the domain of the one who prays alone. Rather it is shared among those who pray and those who receive healing. The gift of healing rests on the intercessors. The gift of healing is imparted to the one who receives that endowment of health through believing praying inspired by the Spirit's Presence.

Most scholars estimate that Jesus spent between six months and a year preaching, teaching, and healing before calling the twelve apostles. Many disciples who began to follow Jesus did so specifically because they witnessed or experienced divine healing; texts like this illustrate Jesus's early ministry:

> *While the sun was setting, all those who had any who were sick with various diseases brought them to Him; and He was laying His hands on each one of them and healing them.* (Luke 4:40)

In fact, it is astonishing to notice how Luke, the physician, speaks of the expectations of the crowds of followers. They didn't merely show up to hear a pleasant word. Most came because they knew that Jesus's teaching was packed with power; they were desperately ill, and they gathered to hear Him with a hope of being healed.

> *Jesus came down with them and stood on a level place; and there was a large crowd of His disciples, and a great multitude of the people from all Judea and Jerusalem, and the coastal region of Tyre and Sidon, who had come to hear Him and to be healed of their diseases; and those who were troubled by unclean spirits were being cured. And all the people were trying to touch Him, because* **power was coming from Him and healing them all.** (Luke 6:17–19)

Power flowed *from* Jesus *to* them.

We are affirming that, just as the woman with the hemorrhage "*felt in her body that she was healed of the affliction*" (Mark 5:29 NKJV), even as Jesus Himself felt a flow of power traveling through Him to accomplish healing, the crowds also did! In fact, many accounts in the Gospels indicate that tangible power flowed from Jesus to them.[11] Long before MRIs, antibiotics, or anesthesia, the sick became well. They came without qualification, recommendation, or status and received healing freely.

Jesus walked in this ministry as *the Word made flesh* and was *God with us.* (See John 1:14; Matthew 1:23.) He was overflowing with compassion for the marginalized, the wounded, the powerless, the weary, and the sick.

---

11. For a small sample, see the following texts: Matthew 14:36; Luke 5:17; Mark 3:10; 5:29–30; 6:56.

What is important for our purposes is to recognize why He did that. It is clearly presented as the pattern of godliness in each of the four Gospels and alluded to in the Acts and in Paul's Epistles. Notice that we are the recipients of a divine gift, an exchange.

In short form:

JESUS, BORN AS A HUMAN, RECEIVED THE POWER OF GOD'S SPIRIT AS A HUMAN SO THAT EVERY HUMAN, BORN OF GOD, MIGHT RECEIVE THE POWER OF GOD'S SPIRIT.

God's purpose in sending Jesus was to grant the gift of God's empowering Presence—Himself—to every human who would receive Him. What a marvelous exchange!

Jesus came to save us. We believe that and embrace it as the foundation of the gospel. Even more importantly:

JESUS CAME TO INFILL AND SATURATE EVERY PORE OF OUR BEINGS WITH HIS SPIRIT! CHRIST CAME TO EMPOWER US WITH THE VERY NATURE, CHARACTER, AND POWER OF GOD.

God's desire is that we do the same works He did, *including entering into praying in the Spirit's power*; in this way, we will see gifts of healing as a part of the ministry of His church all across the earth. Healing prayer is God's idea—not ours. God invented it, and God commands it. Who are we to disobey the God of healing?

This brings us face to face with the issue of the day:

For us to minister as Jesus did, our hearts must receive the power of the Holy Spirit to share and bear God's heart of compassion for the world. The clear language of the *apostle of love* is profoundly moving:

> *Whoever says he abides in him ought to walk in the same way in which*
> *he walked.* (1 John 2:6 ESV)

That John should write this to a church means that John—the last of the original apostles, writing in his old age—expected those early believers to engage in life and ministry using Jesus's methods and approaches to serve as the paradigm for our life in Him.

The apostle John believed that all Jesus's ministry was to continue past the original apostles. There is not even a whisper of a hint that after the death of the original apostles anything would change.

> THOSE TRAINED BY THE LAST ORIGINAL APOSTLE OF JESUS WERE TO DO MINISTRY IN EXACTLY THE SAME WAY AS THE FIRST GENERATION DID.

Jesus did His acts of power through the dynamic power of the Holy Spirit. Part of following Christ in the anointing of the Spirit means praying for sick and suffering people as we cooperate with the movement of God's Spirit in and through us.

We need to see clearly in Scripture that *Healing Prayer is God's Idea for Restoring Body, Mind, and Spirit.* It is plain to read this in His teaching, particularly Jesus's Farewell Discourse recorded in John 14.

> *Truly, truly I say to you, the one who believes in Me, the works that*
> *I do, he will do also; and greater works than these he will do; because*
> *I am going to the Father. And whatever you ask in My name, this I*
> *will do, so that the Father may be glorified in the Son. If you ask Me*
> *anything in My name, I will do it. If you love Me, you will keep My*
> *commandments.* (John 14:12–15)

The text is clear: What He did, we will do!

According to the Lord Himself, we will do even more than He did, as the Holy Spirit anoints His church (the body of Christ) to proclaim the good news of Jesus.

Certainly, the Holy Spirit who empowers us in the work of Christ empowers us for complete identification with Christ.

WE WILL SHARE HIS POWER. WE WILL ALSO SHARE HIS SUFFERING.

Jesus continued:

If the world hates you, keep in mind that it hated me first…They will treat you this way because of my name, for they do not know the one who sent me.   (John 15:18, 21 NIV)

Jesus didn't demonstrate the compassion of God in ideal circumstances, and neither do we. Paul said it beautifully:

Our momentary, light affliction is producing for us an eternal weight of glory far beyond all comparison.   (2 Corinthians 4:17)

Yet most of us have tasted having *our hearts moved with compassion* when someone is ill, distressed, or suffering, whether their affliction is spiritual, mental, emotional, or physical. God deepens our response to that yearning to help within us. He empowers us with His own Spirit— Himself within us—to act in harmony with that longing to want to help, to come alongside the one in trouble, to enter into some of their burden as an intercessor.

In Scripture, a principal signal for Christ to act—and usually to pray in a focused manner—was for His whole being to brim over with compassion. This is exactly what happened when He fed the five thousand. (See Mark 6:34–44.) It's also clearly the case when He met a leper, drained and wearied by grinding despair, who begged that Christ might touch him to heal him.

> Now a leper came to Him, imploring Him, kneeling down to Him and saying to Him, "If You are willing, You can make me clean." Then Jesus, **moved with compassion**, stretched out His hand and touched him, and said to him, "I am willing; be cleansed." As soon as He had spoken, immediately the leprosy left him, and he was cleansed.
>
> (Mark 1:40–42 NKJV)

How do we translate this phrase, *"moved with compassion"*?

PERHAPS WE COULD SAY, "HE BRIMMED OVER WITH A SYMPATHETIC YEARNING FROM DEEP WITHIN," OR "HE WAS UTTERLY MOVED IN THE DEPTHS OF HIS BEING."

It is difficult for our words to adequately capture the intention.

Clearly, God the Son felt emotional anguish in a bond with another that elicited a yearning for that man to be well. For Jesus, praying—and in this case praying for healing—involved *feeling*. It is difficult to carry the plain meaning of the Greek term we translate as *"moved with compassion."*

The intercession began with an emotional yearning for another to be well.

In imitation of the Lord, we find ourselves praying, whether silently or aloud.

Perhaps we groan in anguish as we long for our loved one to be restored. We ask the Lord to intervene, to help, to heal, to save, to make the afflicted one well.

In Scripture, we see the compassion of Jesus rising within Him, prompting His actions. Jesus, who is God incarnate, did not merely or mechanically set about fixing the broken. Rather Jesus *encountered* broken humans in anguish. He *felt* their anguish. Then, being moved internally, He prayed.

That is one form (of many in Scripture) of what is called *"praying in the Spirit."*[12] Here is what that type of praying looked like in the ministry of Jesus:

> GOD'S HEALING GRACE, GOD'S POWER, FLOWED THROUGH AN EMPATHETIC YEARNING, A LOVE-SATURATED PRAYER FOR THE SICK ONE TO BE MADE WELL.

Jesus's ministry of healing arose from God's Spirit and was signaled by His deep yearning that we fallen broken ones be made well.

That Holy Spirit imparted the needed power to accomplish that healing. It is the Holy Spirit who imparts gifts of healing. He also transforms our attitudes and our desires and *transfigures them*, turning our yearning emotions into focused intercession. The Spirit of the Lord grants not only power but also a singular purpose that saturates our praying: we pray in the Spirit as our intercessions are shot through and permeated with the unselfish love of God.

Matthew tells us of Jesus's compassion for the throngs of sick, weary, and wounded souls that caused Him to tell His disciples to pray for God to raise up more workers for the harvest.

> *Jesus was going through all the cities and villages, teaching in their synagogues and proclaiming the gospel of the kingdom, and healing every disease and every sickness. Seeing the crowds,* **He felt compassion for**

---

12. Some believers identify "praying in the Spirit" with "speaking in tongues"—and refer to 1 Corinthians 14:13–19. In that context, the apostle is clearly describing "speaking in tongues" as "praying in the Spirit." Here, Jesus, who did not speak in tongues, was praying as the Holy Spirit intersected and flowed through His entire being. It was an intertwining of His Spirit, the Holy Spirit, and compassion for the afflicted, joined together with human touch. Praying in the Spirit may include tongues or not, as the situation requires.

them, because they were distressed and downcast, like sheep without a shepherd. (Matthew 9:35–36)

After this, Jesus told the disciples to pray for more workers to carry out the ministry that was growing and expanding beyond the limited capacity of a single person. That request included the ministry of healing. Right after Jesus was moved with empathy for the crowds who were sick, suffering, and afflicted, He said:

The harvest is plentiful, but the workers are few. Therefore, plead with the Lord of the harvest to send out workers into His harvest. (Matthew 9:37–38)

Notice the logic: Right after asking them to pray for more workers, Jesus gathered the Twelve to send them out in ministry. (See Matthew 10:1.) They were the first "more workers" in answer to His prayer—and one role they played in this context included praying for the sick.

> WE DON'T OFTEN DRAW THE DOTS CLOSELY ENOUGH: JESUS DID THIS ACTION AS A DIRECT RESULT OF BEING INFILLED BY THE SPIRIT.

In the mind of Jesus of Nazareth, *healing prayer* was God's idea!

He told the new workers to pray with a clear goal in mind—ask God to send even more workers to care for the multiplied thousands of the sick, the lost, the helpless, and the demonized.

In this case, Jesus acted to answer His own prayer, sending His disciples out two by two. Jesus *"gave them authority…to heal every disease and every sickness"* (Matthew 10:1).

Let's be clear: Jesus of Nazareth sent them out as an extension of His ministry. That ministry included a blunt proclamation of the kingdom of God breaking through to this fallen world. Critical to that commissioning was prayer for healing. Here is the command of the Lord to the sending of the Twelve:

> And as you go, preach, saying, "The kingdom of heaven is at hand." Heal the sick, cleanse the lepers, raise the dead, cast out demons. Freely you have received, freely give.   (Matthew 10:7–8 NKJV)

The disciples (strangely, even Judas Iscariot) were sent out with authority to heal, as an extension of Jesus's healing ministry, in direct response to His prayer for more workers to be raised up to heal the sick.

The command of Scripture is to learn from Jesus's methods and apply them.

- ✦ Jesus prayed for the sick.
  - » We should too.
- ✦ Jesus trained teams and taught them to pray for the sick, then sent them out to do the very works He did.
  - » We should too.

Jesus would have us form teams to pray together too, to enter into God's idea of healing prayer. We join our willingness to obey His teaching with the power and compassion of God who equips us with His very own Presence to get this done!

Jesus's mercy on the sick and afflicted people will continue until the close of time. What we have discovered in every church that we have served is that intercessors already know this in their devotions. When drawn into intercession, those who pray actually *feel it with Him*. Here is a clear example from the capital epistle, Romans:

> In the same way the Spirit also helps our weakness; for we do not know what to pray for as we should, but the Spirit Himself intercedes for us with groanings too deep for words.   (Romans 8:26)

The intercessor prays and runs out of words. They groan in wordless anguish, utterly unable to even know how to pray. Then, the Spirit of God Himself joins the praying of the intercessor. They both *feel it*—both groan together: God groans in birthing anguish, and the intercessor groans as God's Spirit prays through them. They are *praying together*! This is so that

God can cause *"all things to work together for good"* (Romans 8:28) through the prayers of God by His Spirit, and the Christ-following intercessor *praying together at the same time.*

When we invite the Holy Spirit to shape our praying, God Himself ignites holy compassion within us. Sometimes God's emotion intersects and redirects ours. This is clearly the point of Paul's teaching on how justification by faith *feels.*

> *Therefore, having been justified by faith, we have peace with God through our Lord Jesus Christ, through whom we also have obtained our introduction by faith into this grace in which we stand; and we celebrate in hope of the glory of God...and hope does not disappoint, because the love of God has been poured out within our hearts through the Holy Spirit who was given to us.*   (Romans 5:1–2, 5)

When we first encounter this amazing grace called *justification*, we feel it. On the level of emotion alone, we receive:

+ Peace with God

+ Exultation in hope

+ Anticipation of participation in glory

+ And, most especially, the love of God—tangibly experienced.

That love is described as something that is "poured out" within our deepest heart by the Holy Spirit.

This is a book about prayer—*Healing Prayer*. It is important to remember that Jesus, enthroned in heaven, didn't stop His work once He rose from the grave. In fact, His greater ministry began as He took His seat in heaven at the place of ruling authority!

He began to rule on His throne!

He rules by praying!

Not only does Jesus live forevermore, but He also pours out His very Spirit, who carries His praying into us and joins us in that magnificent work, and He continues to intercede for us. He invites us now to join Him in His magnificent ministry of healing by surrendering our hearts and hands to Him—our hearts, to be shaped by and filled with His compassion, and our hands, to be available and ready to extend His flowing, healing mercy.

Is the Holy Spirit nudging you to grow in intercession? It most certainly isn't your idea—it's His. *Healing prayer is God's idea.*

REFLECT AND RECORD

1. In this chapter, we have read the apostle John say this: *"Whoever says he abides in him ought to walk in the same way in which he walked"* (1 John 2:6 ESV). This refers to all aspects of the life of Jesus. What might this text be challenging you to do differently?

   _____

   _____

   _____

2. In John 14:12–14, Jesus promises something astonishing—that His disciples will continue His ministry by doing as He did. Read this aloud a couple of times to get it in your thinking.

   Truly, truly I say to you, the one who believes in Me, the works that I do, he will do also; and greater works than these he will do; because I am going to the Father. And whatever you ask in My name, this I will do, so that the Father may be glorified in the Son. If you ask Me anything in My name, I will do it.
   (John 14:12–14)

   Now see if you can "get at" the intention of this text by writing it out in your own words:

   _____

   _____

   _____

3. Do you sense the Holy Spirit putting something in your heart to do *"so that the Father may be glorified in the Son"*? What might that be?

_____

_____

_____

4. Does your deepest desire match the way you are praying? How then should you pray?

_____

_____

_____

A PRAYER TO RECEIVE GOD'S COMPASSION

Lord Jesus, You command us "to walk as You walked," and You tell us to ask for this very thing. So, we ask:

+   *Give me trusting faith to believe that the Holy Spirit can shape my inner being, impart God's love, and empower me to receive Your heart of compassion.*

+   *Anoint me to do Your work with humility, awe, and gratitude.*

In Jesus's name, by Your authority alone, I ask these things. Let it be so in me and in those I love. Amen.

4

MEDICINE, MIRACLE, AND MYSTERY COMINGLE

We didn't know...

We (David and Elizabeth) married with great joy and had no idea that pregnancy could be lethal to my wife. We had no idea she had a genetic liver deficiency, and that rising levels of estrogen in her body during pregnancy would cause her liver to first shut down and then begin to destroy liver tissue.

We married, took a year to settle, and then decided to try for a child. Of course, when the news came that Elizabeth was expecting, our circle of friends and family was delighted. The usual kindnesses began to happen—a baby shower, cards from friends, joyful phone calls from her mom, her sisters, and my family, unexpected gifts...all this and more.

I went to work setting up a room; we got a crib, a car seat, a swing, and clothing. We were getting excited.

Then it happened. Not so serious, just annoying.

Cholestasis of pregnancy.

Itching.

Scratching.

Discomfort.

Sleeplessness.

Yet there was a concerning factor that made us pause: cholestasis usually does not occur until the third trimester. This was Elizabeth's *first* trimester. Then the symptoms grew in frequency and intensity. Annoying became significant, and then became serious.

My wife's skin and eyes began to exhibit jaundice, followed by abnormal bruising.

If I gently touched her arm or tapped her on the shoulder, she developed significant bruising. Elizabeth needed specialists. She drove to one—and he wouldn't let her drive home. She wound up in the perinatal unit of Vancouver Grace Hospital, a teaching hospital that's among the finest in my country, Canada. Two world-class specialists, one in perinatology and the other in hematology, were assigned to her.

Here I must pause for clarity's sake: as Maxie and I continue to teach about healing prayer, let's make something perfectly clear:

WE BELIEVE IN MEDICINE. WE ALSO BELIEVE IN MIRACLE. IN HOLY MYSTERY, MEDICINE AND MIRACLE INTERTWINE.

I (David) have been a pastor for more than thirty years.

My wife and I have witnessed the miraculous—beyond ordinary medicine; we had seen this even before we married, in our first years as friends, and in our early ministry. We have also tasted sadness and loss, as both healing prayer and medical intervention did not yield the hoped-for cure.

What we have *regularly* seen is an intertwining, a joining of the power of God upon the very best of what we know medicine provides. So this chapter will concern itself with an intertwining, a comingling of medicine and miracle.

MEDICINE, MIRACLE, AND ME

With this background clearly in mind, with the knowledge that Elizabeth and I have known the power of the Lord to heal, it is time to return to the account of my wife's health.

She had become more than ill. We were concerned that the child might not live.

So we did what most everyone does when someone is not as they should be. We sought the best medical counsel available—and as believers, we prayed…and prayed…and prayed.

And my wife was not recovering. Her condition got worse.

Three women determined to pray with her, two young moms and a grandma. They would set up a three-way call and seek God with her once a day.

Elizabeth says her body felt like bees were stinging her between her breasts, on the flats of her hands, and on the soles of her feet. Only an ice bath would numb the stings long enough for her to sleep for an hour—and she was growing weaker. Yet when those three women prayed, the stinging would diminish and sometimes cease for five or six hours. This was the only relief Elizabeth experienced apart from the ice baths.

The medical community was baffled and growing increasingly concerned.

So a procedure was booked: an amniocentesis to test for the needed enzymes to indicate lung function in the child. Test completed, the fluid, ordinarily transparent, came out dark green. Our unborn son was swimming in bile and would likely be blind, deaf, and possibly afflicted with cerebral palsy. Additionally, as a result of eroding liver function, Elizabeth's health was failing.

The medical team offered two solutions. At that moment, the pregnancy was thirty weeks along. If she could endure for two more weeks, at thirty-two weeks, they could put her on intravenous medication to induce a "natural" birth. Or they could do a C-section to bring the child out without passing through the birth canal.

There was one issue of concern related to either option: at thirty-two weeks, the lungs of a male baby born prematurely would be barely developed. In those days, surfactant—which coats the lungs to aid early childhood lung development—had just been developed as an experimental drug. It was not known in most hospitals and was most certainly not an ordinary course of action; that meant that if the child's lungs didn't kick-start, there would be a strong possibility of an iron lung on the preemie newborn.

We were more than concerned.

One complicating factor was that I needed to find a new church to serve. I was the associate pastor at a church plant in metro Vancouver—and they couldn't afford two pastors. There was much love there; in fact, decades later, about a dozen of those parishioners showed up for a "great to see you again" visit. Yet the cost of living in metro Vancouver was high—it competes with Toronto as the most expensive city in Canada—and the church was not yet large enough to pay for the rental of a community center, an office, a secretary, and two pastors.

It became clear that I needed to find a new assignment, in the middle of the medical complications of life and death for my wife and unborn child.

There was a church two thousand miles away that was interested in considering me as their lead pastor. Since my wife and son would both be medically compromised, it fell to me to do all I could to provide—and this was the door that opened. And so, in a moment when the liver enzyme levels flattened down to "high but out of danger," I flew to that congregation in Chatham, Ontario, to test out whether we were a match. While I was away, a kind friend named Margo (a friend to this very day) visited Elizabeth in the hospital and stayed nearby in case of emergency.

My first interview on a Sunday evening went well. I was told that I was being given the next morning to pray about the calling, and that a fellow named Bob had offered to drive me around the town in the afternoon, just to get a sense of the area.

It was late July—the hottest time of the year in that community. Temperatures there usually hovered around 90 degrees Fahrenheit for most of July and August—but not on that Monday. It was somewhere between 62 and 65 degrees Fahrenheit,[13] unusually cold for Southwest Ontario. Bob had on a short-sleeve shirt and asked whether I would mind if he stopped at his home to put on some warmer clothing.

After getting the go-ahead, we pulled up at his home, and he invited me inside. He also needed to confirm something with his wife, so I found a chair in the front room and took a seat. Next to the chair was a coffee table with an opened form letter from a medical society.

IT WAS A NEWSLETTER THAT HAD A SHORT, TWO-PARAGRAPH SUMMARY ABOUT THIRTY-TWO-WEEK GESTATIONAL AGE PREEMIE MALES.

The small hairs rose on the back of my neck!

My eyes became glued to that opened form letter.

The note contained a medical synopsis describing the effect of the labor-inducing drip on the emerging child. It said that at thirty-two weeks, the lung development of male preemies would be aided by the pressure of passing through the birth canal. It also said that there was a 35 to 40 percent higher incidence of cerebral palsy because the skull case was soft and underdeveloped. The pressure on the skull could cause the bones to compress too hard on the brain and produce damage that would lead to that syndrome.

After I read the note, Bob and I had our tour, we completed the vetting process, and I was told that I would be recommended to the board and the congregation. I was asked to wait for the congregational vote the next Sunday, and I flew back to Vancouver.

I drove straight to the hospital and met nine physicians as I entered my wife's room. They had been waiting for my arrival, as they needed permissions from both of us to proceed with what they considered to be the best medical solution for my wife's baffling situation.

---

13. Ninety degrees Fahrenheit is 32 degrees Celsius; 62 to 65 Fahrenheit is 16 to 18 degrees Celsius.

All nine of them finally agreed on the approach. They said, "We are going to put Elizabeth on the drip, so that in three days, the child will pass through the birth canal, our best chance to kick-start the lungs." Then they asked if there were any questions.

"Only one!" I said. I paused before continuing.

"Is it not true that with thirty-two-week premature males passing through the birth canal, there is a 35 to 40 percent higher incidence of cerebral palsy as the pressure of the canal on the skull case can cause brain damage?"

Shocked silence filled the room.

Everyone was stunned—my wife, the medical team, *and me*!

I sounded so smart, like I had read reams of current articles on the medical trajectory of male preemies passing through difficult pregnancies! Remember, I had only read two paragraphs from an open form letter in a city two thousand miles away just two days before this.

The doctors looked back and forth at each other as the silence hung in the air. Finally, someone said curtly, "We don't know what to say."

Then all nine left the room while I sat with my wife, expecting a quick return with a trajectory of events. Six hours later, the lead doctor, disheveled and weary, came back into the room. He told us there would be a C-section the following Tuesday. And there was.

Our son, who had been swimming in dark green bile, was born healthy. The physicians had expected him to weigh one to two pounds, but he weighed in at four pounds five ounces—small, but more than viable. He wasn't blind, deaf, or afflicted with cerebral palsy. By a miracle of divine appointment (and not a miracle of healing), we were led to a medical solution, while we prayed with great confusion for a miracle of healing.

There were necessary medical interventions to follow, for both him and Elizabeth—and they were granted. And both are alive to tell the tale.

Years later, we would come to recognize that our son was not impaired during gestation, even though he swam in poison for months. We now believe that this was in fact a miraculous intervention, although we couldn't see that then. A delightful epilogue: at the time of final edits on this manuscript, we celebrated his wedding!

Medicine, miracle, and mystery—their threads of grace intertwine until time ends, and God reveals how those pieces, woven together, comingle to coalesce into a melded tapestry of beauty.

REFLECT AND RECORD

1. Some believe that medicine and miracle are not compatible. What is your view on this tender subject?

_____

_____

_____

2. Second Kings 20 records a moment when a very good king, Hezekiah, was about to die. In fact, God sent a prophet, Isaiah, to tell him. If you read the entire account, you will discover that miracle, prayer, despair, faith, hope, and medicine all played a role. Take a moment to read part of the narrative:

    In those days Hezekiah became ill and was at the point of death. The prophet Isaiah son of Amoz went to him and said, "This is what the LORD says: Put your house in order, because you are going to die; you will not recover." Hezekiah turned his face to the wall and prayed to the LORD, "Remember, LORD, how I have walked before you faithfully and with wholehearted devotion and have done what is good in your eyes." And Hezekiah wept bitterly. Before Isaiah had left the middle court, the word of the LORD came to him: "Go back and tell Hezekiah, the ruler of my people, 'This is what the LORD, the God of your father David, says: I have heard your prayer and seen your tears; I will heal you. On the third day from now you will go up to the temple of the LORD. I will add fifteen years to your life. And I will deliver you and this city from the hand of the king of Assyria. I will defend this city for my sake and for the sake of my servant

David.'" Then Isaiah said, "Prepare a poultice of figs." They did
so and applied it to the boil, and he recovered.

(2 Kings 20:1–7 NIV)

Notice the order of events:

+ Hezekiah became ill

+ God sent Isaiah to tell him to make arrangements for death

+ Hezekiah prayed

+ Isaiah heard God tell him to return. He was required to
  speak a fresh word to the king, that he would live.

+ The prophet had a fig poultice prepared, it was applied to the
  poisoned wound, and the poison went into the poultice so
  that Hezekiah would live!

In the account, there was:

+ *A request from the king for divine proof*

+ *An intercession from the prophet*

+ *A nature miracle—with the terms dictated by the king, and then
  Hezekiah became well after taking his medicine!*

What does this say to us about prayer for healing, medicine,
and miracle?

_____

_____

_____

A PRAYER FOR GUIDANCE

*Dear Lord, medicine, miracle, and mystery intertwine. Yet You ask us
to ask! You ask us to pray and seek You whether we are afflicted or well.
Guide us in our praying and teach us to embrace whatever approach
You send our way—whether the mundane or the miraculous or a mix-
ture that defies explanation but leaves us in awe of who You are! Amen.*

5

WHY WE PRAY FOR HEALING

Through this book, we hope to help you deepen your intercessory life and grow in the practice of praying for healing. We will examine the reasons for *healing prayer* in several sections.

Sometimes healing prayer is fueled by simple desperation: our loved one is in need. And so, we cry out for mercy, grace, love, forgiveness (even when we don't deserve it), and, on the theme of this book, healing.

Prayer also begins with the conviction that if anything is of value, it is the believer's highest choice to turn toward Jesus in our times of deepest need! Simply stated, the truth we have embraced is this affirmation:

PRAYER MATTERS, AND BY THIS GRACIOUS PRACTICE CALLED "INTERCESSION," GOD INVITES US INTO HIS PRESENCE TO PARTNER WITH HIS KINDNESS.

This is stated magnificently in Ephesians:

God, being rich in mercy...made us alive together with Christ...so that in the coming ages he might show the immeasurable riches of his grace in kindness toward us in Christ Jesus. (Ephesians 2:4–5, 7 ESV)

This tells us:

+ God's grace is beyond measure.

+ God's kindness is eternal and can never be exhausted.

Neither God's grace nor God's kindness ever ends. We pray knowing that God's nature is saturated and shot through with grace, revealed in kindness.

Many see prayer as the only thing to do when all hope is lost, after all avenues of healing have been utterly exhausted. Prayer is commonly perceived as something that's main purpose is to prepare a heart for some awful outcome.

MANY SEE PRAYER AS A LAST RESORT OR A WASTE OF TIME. SUCH THINKING IS COMPLETELY ALIEN TO THE CLEAR TEACHING OF THE BIBLE.

Without exception, every leader in Scripture practiced prayer as a primary instrument to accomplish God's calling on their lives—and this included leaders like Moses, Elijah, Samuel the prophet, and, most importantly, none other than Jesus of Nazareth, God the Son.

Jesus is not asking us to waste our time or jump through complicated, intricate hoops in a useless exercise that produces nothing. Rather, if we know how to give good gifts, *"how much more will your Father in heaven give the Holy Spirit to those who ask him!"* (Luke 11:13 NIV).

When we pray for healing, we ask the Holy Spirit to receive our fervent desires for those we love and even those unknown to us whose anguish has come to our attention. To pray for healing is to ask God the Holy Spirit to take our yearnings, place them before Him in an act of surrender, and sift them before the throne of grace. We ask God to inspire us to intercede according to what God knows is best and send discernment to us to pray with the good purposes God holds for the world.

Praying in simple trust yields remarkable fruit beyond our own power—and somehow, some way, miraculously, even though no one deserves it, God intervenes mysteriously and in direct response to our fervent cry!

Praying *alone* produces power.

Praying *together* magnifies that power's effect.

History and current Christian experience together have demonstrated this to be so; prayer's effect is augmented and magnified when the body of Christ cries out together.

In Hebrews 11, a classic text that has been called the "hall of faith," example after example is given of those who were in impossible circumstances. Very often those on that wondrous list were in life-threatening danger. These God-followers sought the Lord in prayer, believing that the very fabric of time and space would be fundamentally altered in a magnificent *reality shift* with God using the sacrifice of their intercessions as the means to reframe reality.

The summary statement says it well:

Without faith it is impossible to please God, *because anyone who comes to him must believe that he exists and that he rewards those who earnestly seek him.* (Hebrews 11:6 NIV)

The key word in this text is *"impossible."* Impossible means that nothing can be done to achieve the desired outcome. Then the writer gives us what is needed to please God:

If you want to please God, the only way is to believe He rewards fervent prayer. Period.

WHY WE PRAY

1. BROKEN WORLD; BROKEN PEOPLE; NEEDING GRACE

Prayer for healing is something God not only welcomes us to practice, He actually commands it! Prayer's effect was built into the fabric of creation. Prayer was and is God's idea. Healing prayer is an extension of one aspect of prayer itself.

Jesus Christ is the Healer for every part of what it means to be human; *"He is before all things, and in him all things hold together"* (Colossians 1:17 NIV). Christ is ready to offer healing to us by mending our broken lives and forgiving our sin. He wants to transform our despair and turn it into a present and future hope, in this life and in the next!

Christ is for us, offering healing in our total being. This includes the realm of the Spirit, the mind, the emotions, and from time to time, as God leads us, in our physical bodies. In *the incarnation* (when God entered creation, and Jesus took on the form of a man), all of human experience was redeemed.

> *EVERY MOLECULE OF JESUS'S HUMAN BODY WAS SATURATED WITH GOD'S SPIRIT. HE DID THAT SO THAT EVERY MOLECULE OF OUR HUMAN BODIES COULD EXPERIENCE THE SAME!*

This is God's antidote for our fallen planet.

Our world is saturated, shot through with sorrow, sin, and death. There is decay, oppression, trauma, grief, pain, and loss. We also find twisted motives within ourselves, and this disturbs us as we find ourselves "whelmed under weight of evil, sick or dead,"[14] our wills bent toward sinning, our loves stunted. The extent of this inner turmoil could seem overwhelming without the power of the grace of God.

Yet through God's sustaining grace, the world is also saturated with the goodness of our Creator. The same grace at work when Jesus was raised from the dead also works in us. When we receive the Holy Spirit, Christ makes us *"partakers of the divine nature"* (2 Peter 1:4)—we become melded together with and joined in fellowship with the Trinity, the Godhead.

---

14. This phrase comes from Dietrich Bonhoeffer's "Letters and Papers from Prison" and is quoted in the hymn "Men Go to God" versified by Walter Henry Farquharson. See Hymn #105 Men God to God, *The Hymn Book of the Anglican Church of Canada and the United Church of Canada*, authorized by General Synod and General Council, 1971.

This means that nothing is out of God's reach. It is in the realm of God's power to make anything and anyone new to the uttermost. Healing prayer is an instrument that God uses to heal our bodies (partially or completely) in this life or to bring that to pass completely in the resurrection life to come.

There is a deeper purpose to healing prayer; this kind of praying finds its best outcome as God shapes us to become like Him. Healing prayer, and all other forms of prayer, have Christlikeness as their ultimate goal. By our praying, we discover that various aspects of the creation are transformed; by the same praying, intercessors are astonished to discover that they are changed as well—"transfigured," or to use the language of the apostle in 2 Corinthians 3:18, *"transformed...from glory to glory."*

We pray about the world, and through that praying, God shapes *us!*

That shaping is the astonishing benefit of seeking God's highest for another. We become like Christ even as the Holy Spirit urges us to pray and to pray for the healing of the sick, soul-weary, and afflicted.

2. THE EXAMPLE OF CHRIST

Do you believe that God invites humans to pray? Well done. The Scripture says that your convictions on this matter are true.

Do you also believe that God has molded the creation to respond to the prayers of people, to change and reshape the world? Here is an astonishing and sobering fact to consider:

Jesus of Nazareth did.

And so, in unity with the Father's desire, Jesus put this into practice in His ministry. Jesus prayed to reshape the earth.

When God became a human in Jesus and *"dwelt among us"* (John 1:14), we discovered something even more profound. Jesus Christ entered into human experience as one of us, only better. He came as "the Second Adam" since the first Adam fell.[15]

---

15. This is the clear intention of Paul's discourse on the resurrection and future hope in 1 Corinthians 15, especially verses 42–49. It is expressed clearly in 1 Corinthians 15:45 (esv), a summary verse: *"Thus it is written, 'The first man Adam became a living being'; the last Adam became a life-giving spirit."*

In that embraced role, Christ repaired our fractured communion with God by practicing communion with God—as a human substitute for us. So how did He do that? It was through the practice of prayer *as the principal occupation of His ministry.*

> *JESUS'S PRAYERS WOULD BE USED BY GOD THE FATHER TO TRANSFORM REALITY.*

When the crowds pressed in to receive His touch, His grace, and His healing, Jesus made sure He did the one thing needed to accomplish the rest: *Jesus prayed—and this was God at prayer!*

Jesus prayed regularly as part of the Jewish framework in which He was raised: Palestinian Jews of the first century would pray a minimum of three times a day, four times on the Sabbath, and as many as seven times a day during holy festivals. The culture He lived in was *prayer saturated.*

Yet Jesus prayed beyond those dedicated daily times, in order to hear the Father's voice and intercede for others. Think about this! That was *God at prayer.*

The continuing ministry of the risen and ascended Christ is a ministry of intercession. Regardless of whatever gifts of the Spirit you may have (or not have), every follower of Jesus Christ is called to join Him in that ministry. In the epistle to the Hebrews, it is powerfully expressed:

> *Because Jesus lives forever, he has a permanent priesthood. Therefore he is able to save completely those who come to God through him, because* **he always lives to intercede for them.** (Hebrews 7:24–25 NIV)

If Jesus *"always lives to make intercession"* (Hebrews 7:25), then those who want to know Christ and spend time with Him will join Him in doing exactly the same thing. To know Christ is to join Him in praying—certainly that same call is upon us.

As we have seen in chapter 3, after noting that creation groaned because it was not as it should be and that believers groaned because they were not as they should be (see Romans 8:22–23), Paul wrote of his experience of the Spirit while praying. He says that God by His Spirit groans because the creation and believers are not as they should be: *"The Spirit Himself intercedes for us with groanings too deep for words"* (Romans 8:26).

If we understand that the Spirit is in fact a part of the Godhead, then when we pray, we become merged with and participate in the life of the Trinity through the Spirit's ministry of prayer.

WHEN THE SPIRIT PRAYS WITH US, FOR US, OR THROUGH US, THIS IS, ONCE AGAIN, GOD AT PRAYER!

Prayer for healing is an extension of the ongoing ministry of the risen Lord. This ministry does not belong to any one person; it belongs to God, and through God's invitation, we join in God's grace at work.

Remember this: Jesus's work did not end with the cross. Rather, it was launched on the cross, was magnified by the resurrection and ascension, and now expands across all time and space as more and more believers are brought into the fullness of God's Spirit.

As those joined to Christ, we participate in all that is of Christ Himself. We actually enter into His intermediary role, this ministry called *the priesthood*. This scriptural treasure, the "priesthood of all believers," helped spark the fires of the Protestant Reformation. (See 1 Peter 2:9–10.)

You are a priest, and so are we!

What do priests do?

+ Priests *speak to God* for the people—that is intercession
+ Priests *speak to people* with the good news of Christ, testifying of what we know of Him in word, deed, and sign

Behind every form of ministry, including prayer for healing, believers join with Jesus's ministry through the transforming power of the Holy Spirit.

3. THE FAITH PASSED DOWN

History is clear; often, the revival of the church has come in the wake of *signs and wonders*. It was certainly true of the Methodist revival in eighteenth-century England. Besides the practical things that John and Charles Wesley developed—such as organizing people to learn and pray together in small and medium-sized groups and teaching basic disciplines—the far-reaching impact the Wesleys had was primarily the result of the supernatural Presence and power of the Holy Spirit in the revival meetings, the small groups, and in their preaching.

Unusual signs, manifestations of power, and remarkable healings were a regular part of John Wesley's ongoing ministry. In a letter to Conyers Middleton, Wesley described how he understood various gifts of the Spirit. That letter was drafted to defend the teaching that every gift of the Spirit named in the Bible continued through church history to present day.[16]

Testimony to the power of the Holy Spirit continued in the movements that arose in North America in the eighteenth and nineteenth centuries. Despite the sordid and mixed history of racism that divided American church movements, new expressions of Christ's body were formed. These new bodies bore witness to the power of the Holy Spirit. In the fires of revivalism in the 1800s, Thomas Doty recounted that African Methodist Episcopal (AME) Zion evangelist Julia Foote "held the almost breathless attention of five thousand people, by the eloquence of the Holy Ghost, [we] know well where is the hiding of her power."[17] Rev. Foote, writing about newly integrated meetings of Methodists in Zanesville, Ohio, testified with these words:

God the Holy Ghost was powerfully manifest in all meetings. I was the recipient of many mercies. In all of them I could trace the

---

16. For a modern paraphrase on Wesley's views on the Holy Spirit, see John Wesley, *The Holy Spirit and Power*, paraphrased by Clare Weakley (Plainfield, NJ: Logos International, 1977), especially 81–94, in which Weakley demonstrates Wesley's defense of the Spirit's gifts from the early church and the New Testament. See also Wesley's "Letter to Dr. Conyers Middleton," January 4, 1749.

17. Julia A. J. Foote, *A Brand Plucked from the Fire: An Autobiographical Sketch* (Wilmore, KY: First Fruits Press, 2019), 7.

hand of God and claim divine assistance whenever I most needed it. Whatever I needed, by faith I had. Glory! Glory!! While God lives, and Jesus sits at his right hand, nothing shall be impossible unto me, if I hold fast faith with a pure conscience.[18]

After preaching one Sunday evening in Albany, New York, she testified that, "the entire audience seemed moved to prayer and tears by the power of the Holy Ghost."[19]

The nineteenth-century holiness movement, sparked from the fires of Wesleyan Methodism, inspired other movements that witnessed to the power of the Holy Spirit. The Christian and Missionary Alliance (C&MA) arose after its founder, Presbyterian Albert Benjamin Simpson, experienced a personal infilling of the power of the Holy Spirit and was granted a remarkable healing. He went from being sickly and unable to carry out a program of visitation in his local church to traveling to more than sixty nations, climbing mountain passes, and traversing treacherous pathways—and he did this before aviation or cars were common.

He actually planted a church in Mongolia!

Simpson proclaimed a summary of his gospel that is still required of anyone in the movement: the "fourfold gospel" of the C&MA upholds that Jesus is "Savior, Sanctifier, Healer, and Coming King." Simpson and those who joined him in the early Alliance saw signs and gifts of the Spirit catapult his fledgling mission's society into some of the least-reached regions of the planet, which now themselves send out workers in multiple directions.

The many branches of Wesleyan Methodism, along with denominations like the C&MA, influenced American Pentecostalism, which embraced Simpson's fourfold gospel and added the necessity of various sign gifts.[20] These streams, among many others, circle the earth with a

---

18. Ibid., 103.
19. Ibid., 92.
20. In fact, one Pentecostal denomination, the international Foursquare Church founded by Aimee Semple McPherson, uses a logo that's almost identical to C&MA's. Semple studied at Simpson College, learned Simpson's fourfold emphasis, and eventually taught that Jesus is the Savior, the Spirit-Baptizer, the Healer, and the Coming King. Its most recent exemplar, the late Jack Hayford, had a similar trajectory. He began in the C&MA, embracing Simpson's fourfold gospel, and eventually became a strong internationally recognized leader in the Foursquare.

gospel that beats with the heart of the Holy Spirit. Yet long before these streams emerged in church history, the power of the Holy Spirit could be found from settings as unique as the ministry of Saint Patrick to the Irish, all the way back to the Spirit sending Philip to explain Isaiah 53 and the gospel of Jesus Christ to an Ethiopian eunuch who was reading while in his chariot. (See Acts 8:26–39.)

The power of the Holy Spirit shows up again and again throughout the family tree of the Christian faith, even in broken branches or when it seemed that the weight of corruption must surely get the last word. But God's grace cannot be contained. Christians long before us have prayed with profound depth, and many have prayed for and witnessed healing.

4. CREATED FOR COMMUNION

If you have ever wondered at the power of prayer, consider this:

Prayer is God's idea.

When we pray, we are responding to God, in partnership with Christ our high priest, who sends the anointing of the Holy Spirit. There is nothing more astonishing than this:

> OUR INTERCESSION BECOMES JOINED TO THE INTERCESSION OF JESUS.

And so, we approach prayer with joy, not reluctance. We know that when we pray, we are living out the reality of being joint heirs with Christ, participants in God's kingdom enterprise. In God's dealing with us, God has made our praying a genuine means to change us and to change our world. Through prayer, God accomplishes the plans of His grace, in individuals and in our towns and cities.

God calls us to join in as *go-betweens* in prayer. God has so shaped the earth that our prayers—yours and mine—have become a primary channel through which God is at work in the world today, rebuilding the brokenness of the world into beauty.

We remember the word of Archbishop Richard C. Trent: "We must not conceive prayer as an overcoming of God's reluctance, but a laying hold of God's highest willingness."

Pastor Shalom Liddick speaks to us on the nature of intercession:

Remember: you are your brother's keeper; you are your sister's keeper. You're a watchman. And where God has placed you, God has placed you on purpose. Watchmen stand in the middle, to communicate, to see, to defend. An intercessor stands in the middle to intervene on behalf of somebody else. The word "intercessor" is a word of the courtroom. Intercessory prayer is prayer given up to God when you stand in the middle to intervene for somebody else. God calls me and calls you to be people who get in the middle and say, "God, can you help my sister? Can you help my brother? Can you help my community?"[21]

Consider these examples from Scripture:

+   God will bless Elijah and send rain, but Elijah must pray for this to happen. (See 1 Kings 18:1.)

+   If God's chosen nation is to prosper, Samuel must plead. (See 1 Samuel 7:8.)

+   If the Jews are to be delivered, Esther must fast and advocate. (See Esther 4:15–16.)

+   God entered the human race in Jesus Christ to heal us, yet Jesus must pray. (See, for example, Luke 5:15–16.)

God invites us—as humans made in God's image, made new by God's grace—to imitate Him in what we do with the life we are given. Prayer is genuine participation in the universe created and sustained by God, effecting real change, confident in the grace of God that works out God's redemptive purposes in the world.

---

21. Shalom Liddick, "Your Brother's Keeper, Sister's Keeper: Intercessory Prayer," February 1, 2020, retrieved March 2021, *Wesleyan Accent*, wesleyanaccent.com/shalom-liddick-your-brothers-keeper-sisters-keeper-intercessory-prayer.

We are called into communion and intercession in prayer; we have the invitation to respond in trust, available to see the unfolding of the grace of Jesus Christ in our own lives and the lives of others.

> *PRAYER DOES NOT LIMIT THE POWER AND SOVEREIGNTY OF GOD; IT IS A VIBRANT MEANS ORDAINED BY GOD THROUGH WHICH GOD'S GRACE UNFOLDS. GOD USES THE PRAYING OF THE FAITHFUL TO RESHAPE REALITY.*

While there may be seasons in which we have not discerned God's will in every area of life, Jesus still urges us to pray, emboldening us to pray confidently.

If you remain in Me, and My words remain in you, ask whatever you wish, and it will be done for you.   (John 15:7)

While we may not always know exactly what to pray, we can always focus on remaining in Christ. We can memorize the words of Jesus, speak with Him about what they mean, and ponder them as we pray. This sets up the conditions for answered prayer and prepares us to pray for the healing of lost cultures as well as healing of the sick, traumatized, and afflicted. It also frees us from focusing on ourselves, our doubts, and our limitations. This opens an important door for the outflowing of God's Presence and power.

As you will see, believing prayer led to the healing of a prison—and it can be *"for the healing of the nations"* (Revelation 22:2).

A TESTIMONY: PRAYER THAT TRANSFORMS A COMMUNITY

In ways that are mysterious and hopeful, God has chosen prayer as a means of change, healing, redemption, and reconciliation. I (Maxie) keep a visible reminder of this in a prominent place where my wife and I pray together most mornings. Displayed where I can easily see it is a wood carving of praying hands. The inscription on it reads, "*The Hands of the Carpenter: Jesus Intercedes for Us (Heb. 7:25)*."

That wood carving of praying hands is a gift from Jeannine Brabon, a longtime missionary in Medellin, Colombia. The hands were carved by Carlos Velasquez, who was a prisoner in Bellavista prison and was converted as a result of prayer baptizing that prison.

Bellavista had been one of the worst prisons in all of Latin America. It was built to house 1,500 inmates. Instead, 5,000 were packed into it like packaged bundles of human flesh.

Until a few years ago, it was a hell pit of violence and inhumanity. Prisoner rape was common, heads were cut off and kicked about like soccer balls, and suicides averaged a staggering fifty per month. It takes little imagination to cringe at the thought. Hell-on-earth is an apt description.

Then something happened.

The story is found in David Miller's book, *The Lord of Bellavista*.[22]

Oscar Osorio, one of the prisoners kept there, had a vision of God wrapping His arms around the prison and taking it in His hands. Osorio received a distinct call to prayer, with a clear divine impression to raise white flags outside the cell block where prayer was taking place.

And so, those inmates who were bold enough to believe that God could change that sordid nightmare began to gather, of all things, to pray together—to intercede for God to move in a prison characterized by violent murder, rape, betrayal, hopeless despair, and suicide.

It did not seem that much happened at first, but those prisoners kept praying, inviting anyone who wanted to join them in prayer, posting the white flag each time they prayed.

It took six long, slow years.

They prayed fervently while surrounded by egregious violence in overcrowded conditions that would make most hearts quail with despair.

But after six years of faithful intercession, Christian conversion began to replace suicide. Where there had been fifty suicides a month, there was now on average only one an entire year—all because Oscar Osorio and a

22. David Miller, *The Lord of Bellavista* (London: Triangle/SPCK Publishing, 1998).

band of Christians responded to God's call to prayer. Prayer groups were established in every cell block. A secular jurist reported that violence in the prison diminished by 90 percent.

Carlos, who carved my set of praying hands, was one of the many converts. Now released from prison, he travels in the United States and throughout Latin America, witnessing to the Lord of Bellavista, the vital force of prayer, and how the Lord transformed his life and that hellish prison.

WHY DO WE PRAY FOR HEALING?

To pray is to experience the reality that prayer is far more than just a last resort before we throw in the towel. Prayer is a gift to be embraced, the means by which God reshapes our fallen, hurting planet. God invites our genuine participation in prayer; by God's grace, our prayers make a difference in our world—just like Jesus's prayers did. Through the prayers of His people, God's grace calls and redeems lost souls, reshapes corrupt cultures, turns the hearts of leaders, rewrites the stories of nations, and softens hardened extremists into joyful saints. Consider how the murderous, hate-saturated Saul became the apostle Paul, who wrote, *"Love is patient, love is kind..."* (1 Corinthians 13:4).

In short, God takes your prayer and uses it to transform our world to become more like His kingdom. Whether your words are eloquent or you can barely string two words together, it doesn't matter: God invites everyone to bring their deepest joys or griefs, on their best days or in their worst moments.

Praying by ourselves holds significant power. Jesus prayed alone to focus, hear, and intercede.

PRAYING FERVENTLY ALONE RELEASES GOD'S POWER. PRAYING FERVENTLY TOGETHER MAGNIFIES GOD'S POWER TO RESHAPE THE WORLD.

Praying with others—concerted, focused praying—magnifies the effect of that intercession. Jesus took His three closest disciples (Peter, James, and John) with Him for significant times of prayer—the transfiguration, the raising of Jairus's daughter, and the garden of Gethsemane.

REFLECT AND RECORD

1. God created the world to respond to and be remade through prayer. He made prayer to communicate with Him. Jesus Christ, fully God and fully human, practiced regular prayer. Do you have a time or place to pray? Are there hurdles to your desire to grow in prayer?

_____

_____

_____

2. Jesus made prayer His regular and frequent priority, putting it ahead of everything else. Is it tempting to want certain outcomes guaranteed before investing time and practice in the discipline of prayer?

_____

_____

_____

3. Oscar Osario started a prayer meeting in a wretched prison. It took six years to prevail, but prevail they did. A vision of Christ in the midst of horrific evil was the motivator. What might that mean for your praying?

_____

_____

_____

A PRAYER TO EMBRACE PRAYING WITH JOY

Jesus, You knew it was more than important for You to pray. It was Your very life, Your ministry. You prayed before healing or teaching. We confess we have not always made prayer the priority in our own lives. You know the distractions, hurdles, or wounds that inhibit drawing near to You. The Holy Spirit is eager to join our praying to Yours! Let prayer be our joy and a gift, not merely a duty. Lord, teach me to pray first, last, and at every opportunity over everything in between. Give us a glimpse of the delight You take in our company, before You ever send us out to serve Your kingdom. Let it be, now, in this moment. Amen.

6

THE SPIRIT PRAYED THROUGH ME

COMPASSION'S SIGNAL AND HEALING BY SURPRISE

If you read of the ministry of Jesus closely, you will soon discover that God sent Him signals to pray.

We have already noted that He and the crowds felt healing power flow. One of the significant signals in the ministry of Jesus and for us is an other-centered yearning for another to be well. This yearning enters into the emotional core of a person to lead them into prayer for healing.

We said this in chapter 3 when referring to the moment when Jesus prayed for a leper to be healed in Mark 1:40–41. Rising compassion was common in the ministry of Jesus.

This God-honoring longing for another to be well could be a prompting from the Lord. Clearly, in Jesus's earthly ministry, it was a significant indicator for Him.

When we find ourselves moved by compassion, it may well be that *something is afoot*—that God the Spirit may be inviting us to intercede. It isn't always the case. There are many who simply desire what is best for anyone they meet. Yet should that emotion rise within us unexpectedly, the first thing we should do is to ask whether God might be behind that prompting. The question is whether this invitation will be examined and embraced when the signal shows up—even in times when everything seems utterly inconvenient.

This happened to me (David) while I was going about my ordinary duties as a pastor of a local church in Southwestern Ontario. I was caught completely off guard—and in time, it became clear that God planned it that way.

Gifts of healing can catch us by surprise. They are granted when we least expect them. That is the case with this account.

The man was seventy-two, six foot three, with a straight back and a full head of red-gray hair. He had a muscled torso, even in his senior years. Ron was retired military, having served in World War II and the Korean War. He had worked at his health all of those years after his service. He regularly attended church and consistently sat in exactly the same place, holding hands with his wife, Marion, who was maybe five feet tall when she wore her heels and was thin enough to make most models mildly envious.

They always held hands in public, and in that town of forty thousand or so, I often saw them out for a walk together, chatting and doting on each other post-retirement.

One late-September day, they called for a lovely reason: the fellow wanted to know if I would perform a service of blessing for their fiftieth wedding anniversary the following spring. Those kinds of calls don't require much thinking!

"Of course," I said. "Wild horses couldn't keep me away from a special time like that!"

We pulled out our calendars and locked the day for the occasion.

"Do you want me to drop by quickly to firm up the planning?" I asked.

"Take your time, pastor," the man replied. "We have a date set up, so we can send out the invitations. We'll invite you over for cake and coffee soon."

About a month later, in late October, the couple asked me over for the visit.

Now there are times when a pastoral call consists of showing up, sitting down, and having a chat and a prayer. There are other times when it quickly becomes clear that the visit requires *best foot forward* and formal manners. This time, it was the latter. This couple was *old school* and wanted a visit with the pastor.

I arrived with my planner for notes and was ushered into the dining room. The table was laid out, adorned with a lace tablecloth, a silver tea service, and different types of cakes and muffins on *the good china*. The man seated me on one side of the table across from his wife, and he settled himself into the head chair. The lady asked if she could pour out either tea or coffee, and so began the visit.

After a few minutes of serving cakes and tea, the fellow asked whether I had brought my planner with me.

"Of course!" I replied. "This is our time to write down some thoughts about a solid tribute to fifty years of marriage."

Ron spoke directly to me. "Marion and I were wondering whether you would be able to change the date to sometime between Christmas and the New Year?"

I quickly pulled out my planner (we used paper in those days). There were two days clear just before my post-Christmas holiday, so we circled one of them and got back to the work of planning.

"Are you saving money for your family, so that they don't have to travel twice, once for Christmas and the other for the anniversary?" I asked.

Marion started to softly weep as Ron fixed his gaze on me.

"No," he said. "I will be dead by the spring."

After a pause, the old soldier continued, "I have just been told that I have stage 4 bone cancer, and it is inoperable. The doctor has given me four to six months to live; we believe that I can be well enough in December to celebrate fifty years with the woman I have loved for all these years."

He said this in a matter-of-fact manner, his face completely calm. He had served in two wars and had settled his eternity decades before; those wars required that this be faced before the battles.

"I am at peace with God, my financial affairs are in order, my business is sold, our home is debt-free, the children are raised and well launched, our family has a nest egg, so Marion will be able to continue with her needs taken care of…"

On he spoke, in an undistracted manner. The man chatted from the perspective of complete peace about his eternity. Of course, my jaw was now ajar. I have a vague, foggy memory of dropping my pen, and my eyes becoming unfocused. I was expecting a conversation about a joyful anniversary, not an agonizing death from the slow encroachment of cancer.

He continued. "Now write this down. Here are the Scriptures I want you to read at my funeral…"

He alternated between telling me what he wanted for the anniversary and what should happen once he died. It was almost surreal, listening to a man plainly chat about death and dying while his lovely wife Marion was doing her best to keep *a stiff upper lip* even as the tears were rolling down her cheeks. I was unable to focus in those first few minutes as I processed what this man was saying.

"I will soon be dead," he said.

He would soon have an anniversary service, he said.

Ron told me that I would do both services—they had planned this before I arrived that day. So, the matter settled in his mind, Ron proceeded with his planning:

"Here is the best way to do this service, pastor… Here are the Scriptures. This is my favorite hymn—use this at the close of the funeral. Maybe we should use this during the anniversary too…?"

Even as my emotions were reeling, something started to happen deep within my interior being.

It began as an interior sensing—a gentle fire, rising peace, a conviction of hope, merging with a growing sense of compassion. This turned into a yearning, birthed from within my deepest heart, to ask the Lord to extend His hand to heal.

I had closed my eyes to orient myself to what I had just learned, to absorb the shock and likely stop the tears from flowing for this lovely family, who were kind, gentle, and consistent in their walk with God. As I closed those eyes of mine to gain perspective, a picture quietly floated up from my spirit and settled into the eye of my imagination. That image/ picture surfaced and settled into my mind's eye as the fiery Presence grew within. It was as if I *saw* an image of me reaching my right hand around the back of this man's head, resting it just over his right ear. Then there was an interior compulsion within, a prompting to pray that God would grant this seventy-two-year-old man a healing from the inoperable cancer.

I looked over at him and asked this question in a gentle manner: "May I pray for you?"

The man paused, sat back, and looked at me.

After a moment, he straightened his back, squared his shoulders, and said, "I am at peace with God. My two children are raised. Our finances are in order. Our mortgage is paid off…"

It was clear. Anyone in the ministry for more than a year knows that his answer was understated code. It meant, "Pastor, no. My time has come. And don't ask again."

Then Ron went back to describing what should be done in those two services. Yet my spirit and mind were both blanking out on his words.

The fiery Presence within grew larger. It was as if my heart had grown larger to contain a combination of compassion, fire, and now flowing power. My right hand began to tingle, and the picture in my mind's eye became focused and crystal clear. And so, I asked again.

"May I pray for you?"

Remember, this man was retired military, and judging by external appearance, he was in great shape. He straightened up a second time, looming large over the dinner table. He took hold of the edges of the table-top and raised his voice a notch higher than when he'd responded to my question the first time. The words were the same, but there was an edge to them this time. I wondered if he thought I had missed basic training for pastors. He said, "I am at peace with God. My two children are raised. Our finances are in order. Our mortgage is paid off…"

Then he looked sternly at me. There was no verbal rebuke, but the implication was, "And if you didn't get it the first time, don't ask again." He returned to speaking about the planning for the two services, one a celebration of joy and the other an end to a life lived before God.

Yet I couldn't hear what he was saying—I was utterly unable to focus externally as the interior of my being became consciously aware of a growing sense of Presence.

That fiery Presence filled my whole being; my heart was pounding, and I no longer had to close my eyes to see a picture of me placing my right hand just over and around his right ear.

I asked a third time.

The man looked visibly upset.

So, I asked a fourth time, barely able to stop myself from proceeding with the prayer without his permission—something no one should do.

He stared at me the fourth time and asked in a blunt, rigid rejoinder, "Why are you asking me these four times if you can pray for me when I have told you a clear '*no*' these last three times?"

Finally, gently, I said, "I believe that the Lord is asking me to pray for you to be healed of that cancer, so that you can bring joy to your wife of fifty years and to your family. There is yet work for you to do here."

The man paused at the mention of his wife and an assignment from God for his last days. Her jaw had dropped, and she was staring at me as I spoke those words. Then she looked at him and gave a gentle nod. That nod was her nonverbal assent to my prayer; words are hardly needed when a couple has been married just about fifty years.

He nodded back. He looked at me as if he had to accommodate the pastor's need to pray, and he said, "Well, you're the pastor. Go ahead."

Then he added, "But I'm married fifty years. I am at peace with God. My two children are raised. Our finances are in order. Our mortgage is paid off..."

I reached across before he changed his mind. My right hand was now tingling and burning with heat, and I placed that hand over his right ear.

Suddenly, "Presence" filled the room.

There are no words to describe it.

It was like we were inhaling compassion.

Marion began to weep—but this time, they were tears of yearning, of hope. Ron, who had been agitated and upset at my repeated asking, visibly relaxed as the prayer began. He felt "fiery love," an apt description for God's healing power, course into his body. Every muscle in his frame became completely at ease. He rested his head on the lace tablecloth and muttered a question as he realized that God was at work within him.

"What is that fiery heat flowing into my body, coursing all through me?" he asked.

"That is the Presence of God the Holy Spirit. Christ has sent His Spirit to touch the afflicted areas of your body," I said with confidence and gentle conviction.

After a pause, he said, "Keep praying."

And so, we did—Marion, Ron, and I. We kept praying for as long as we felt that fiery Presence.

I cannot tell you how long that lasted.

You don't look at the clock when you are in the midst of a manifestation of the Spirit's power. You only become conscious of one thing alone—that God is at work, and in holy mystery, Jesus is at work sending His Spirit to flow through you. As in the account of the woman with the issue of blood, all of us felt *the flow of power*. (See Mark 5:29–30.)

Then that Presence *lifted*, leaving a sense of gentle peace and internal consolation.

All three of us knew we were done at exactly the same moment. The prayer was completed—yet we were still aware of the Presence surrounding us and filling us.

We were drawn toward and into a sense of *resting peace*—something of the Lord's grace, directly after that sense of *Manifest Presence at work* was completed.

After a moment, Ron went to a couch in the front room and decided to stay there. He still felt that interior fire coursing through him. This story predates cell phones, so I gave him the numbers for my home and the church and told him to call anytime he had a question.

A few days later, when I was out on a different visit, he called my home and spoke to my wife. "Why is it that every time I read the Bible or pray, that fiery heat courses through my body again?" he asked.

"God is testifying to you that He is at work within your body," my wife replied.

Later we learned that this experience of a sense of interior fire lasted for weeks. Any time the man prayed, read the Bible, or took part in a worship service, he would sense that fiery Presence concentrated in various areas within his body.

After our prayer time, Ron and Marion let the matter rest, as they followed through with all the medical advice that they had received.

A few weeks later, on a Thursday morning, my administrative assistant walked into my office. I was putting the finishing touches on the Sunday sermon. Now, she had been invited to Ron and Marion's anniversary celebration. She knew about his cancer, the spring date, and the Christmas season event.

"Ron and Marion called. They have insisted they need to see you immediately." Linda looked at me with a fixed gaze.

We locked eyes.

Before I could ask, she said, "I will cancel your other appointments for today."

I got into the car and drove right over to their house.

Their table was set with a lace tablecloth, the silver tea service, and pastries and muffins on the good china for the pastor. I was ushered into *exactly* the same spot. Once again, Marion asked if she could *pour out* the tea.

Then, after we all had treats on our plates, Ron looked at me. Locking his eyes on mine, he said, "Had a biopsy done."

He paused.

"Got the results back early this morning."

He stopped. He looked at Marion and then at me.

"Cancer is gone!" he said.

Then, after a pause, he nodded his head, gave an enormous wink with a head nod, and said, "We know who got that!"

That was Ron and Marion's conservative way of saying, "Praise God! Hallelujah."

It was then that they told me that the cancer had been concentrated just above his ear on his right side, and that the fiery Presence at work within continued for weeks.

As you can well imagine, our visit was magical. We shared much from our deepest hearts. When the visit was over, we offered up thanks to Christ the Healer. I did in fact have the privilege of celebrating the blessing of their fifty years of marriage at the anniversary service. The gathered crowd of family and longtime friends heard the testimony of the Lord's power to heal.

There is an epilogue to this account.

Years later, I was teaching a one-week intensive course at a training institute for my denomination. After I told the story to the class, a student raised his hand and asked if he could speak. I gave him permission, and the young fellow said:

> My name is Tyler. I have heard that story before. You see, that was my grandfather in that story. I was doing shift work and was sleeping there because their home was quiet. I stepped out after you left. My grandfather told me exactly the same story. He told me that you had come over and prayed for him. He said that he felt a fiery heat coursing through his body and that you had told him Jesus was healing him. That was the beginning of my call to Christ and then my call to be a pastor.

The class marveled at the story when I told it—and then they were all astonished when Tyler asked to speak and verified the account from *the other side*. You see, they knew him and discovered that there was a living witness to the account I told—someone they knew as a colleague and classmate.

Ron lived nine more years and passed away at age eighty-one of something else altogether. His wife passed shortly after that. They were both given a gift of grace—a gift of love from Christ our Lord. None of us—not me, Ron, Marion, or their grandson Tyler, sleeping down the hall—had anticipated that these events would happen.

It was not our idea.

It was "healing by surprise."

And when the signal was given, *being moved with compassion*, joined with a growing of the divine Presence, and married to a clear conviction to pray in real time, we cooperated with the divine Presence. Together we *embraced God's invitation to intercede* because *healing prayer is God's idea*.

REFLECT AND RECORD

1. This healing prayer account concerns an event that caught everyone by surprise. God *interrupted their day!* When you read the Bible, it quickly becomes clear that God acted this way with many. For example, Peter, James, and John were called when they were out fishing. (See Luke 5:1–11.) Have you ever found yourself in the middle of a *God moment* when you were completely surprised? Describe that.

   _____

   _____

   _____

2. Mark 5 contains several accounts of divine healing—a demonized man set free, a woman with a hemorrhage being healed, and the daughter of Jairus raised from the dead. Each one included the element of surprise. One refers to an experience in which Jesus and an unnamed woman "*felt*" a flow of power. Take a moment to read of her healing:

   A woman who had had a hemorrhage for twelve years, and had endured much at the hands of many physicians, and had spent all that she had and was not helped at all, but instead had become worse—after hearing about Jesus, she came up in the crowd behind Him and touched His cloak. For she had been

saying to herself, "If I just touch His garments, I will get well."
And immediately the flow of her blood was dried up; and **she**
felt in her body that she was healed *of her disease. And imme-*
diately Jesus, **perceiving in Himself that power from Him**
had gone out, *turned around in the crowd and said, "Who*
touched My garments?" And His disciples said to Him, "You
see the crowd pressing in on You, and You say, 'Who touched
Me?'" And He looked around to see the woman who had done
this. But the woman, fearing and trembling, aware of what had
happened to her, came and fell down before Him and told Him
the whole truth. And He said to her, "Daughter, your faith has
made you well; go in peace and be cured of your disease."

(Mark 5:25–34)

What did the woman *feel*?

_____

_____

_____

What did Jesus *feel*?

_____

_____

_____

Have you ever *felt* the Presence of God? What did that feel like?

_____

_____

_____

3. Make a commitment to pay attention to rising compassion. It could be something as ordinary as you responding to someone else's distress. However, it could be God sending a word to you, via your emotional bond with Christ, that you are to pray for another.

_____

_____

_____

A PRAYER TO RESPOND TO THE PRESENCE

Lord Jesus, You were present to the Presence whenever You prayed. You felt tangible power flow through You, often when you felt compassion. So, Lord, use me any way You choose—and if You choose to make me aware of Your action by moving on me with a tangible sense of power, or a rising sense of compassion for another, grant that I cooperate to see Your work done. Amen.

7

THE INDWELLING CHRIST: A FORGIVING AND HEALING PRESENCE

Presence of God in Jesus Christ is not to be experienced only on occasion; rather, the indwelling Christ is to be the guiding and shaping power of our lives. This assertion is at the core of my (Maxie's) theology and the call upon my life as a Christian.

I believe there are two central experiential concepts in Christian theology: one, *justification by grace through faith*, which is our theology of salvation; and two, *the indwelling Christ*, which defines the nature and source of power for Christian living. He indwells us by the Presence of His Spirit.

Justification by grace through faith has always been central in Protestant Christianity and is now increasingly embraced by all branches of His church. Yet this second concept, the understanding of Christians living as persons being *alive in Christ*, has been grossly ignored. For that reason, we have anemic expressions of Christianity. We have reduced faith in Christ to a dry belief system, doctrinal statements to which we ascribe, and creeds that we repeat out of rote memory, but do not affirm experientially. The radical notion of New Testament Christianity is just this:

The promise of the gospel is that what Jesus did during His earthly life and ministry, He continues to do as God's living Presence in our world today. What He said then were eternal words; those words have the same probing, judging, comforting, and guiding power for us today.

What He was, He still is.

PRESENCE OF GOD IN JESUS CHRIST IS NOT TO BE EXPERIENCED ONLY ON OCCASION; RATHER, THE INDWELLING CHRIST IS TO BECOME THE SHAPING POWER OF OUR LIVES.

You and I, through faith, can experience Him in vital Presence and dynamic power, in just the same way as those who knew Him in the flesh in ancient Galilee.

It is essential that we claim this truth in our praying, especially when we are called to healing prayer. The prayer of Paul in Ephesians 3 is to be answered in the life of every Christian: *"That you may be filled to **all the fullness of God"** (Ephesians 3:19).*

All the fullness of God! How can that be?

It is a gift, measureless grace, available to each of us. Paul wrote about the means by which this is accomplished:

I pray that out of his glorious riches he may strengthen you with power through his Spirit in your inner being, so that Christ may dwell in your hearts through faith. And I pray that you, being rooted and established in love, may have power, together with all the Lord's holy people, to grasp how wide and long and high and deep is the love of Christ, and to know this love that surpasses knowledge—that you may be filled to the measure of all the fullness of God. (Ephesians 3:16–19 NIV)

How that is to happen is clear: It is by Christ dwelling in our hearts in love, His Spirit within us. This understanding and cultivation of the indwelling Presence of Christ is crucial to our life as Christians and is especially important to our intercessory praying.

In writing to the Colossians, Paul called this *the mystery.*

Now I rejoice in my sufferings for your sake, and in my flesh I am supplementing what is lacking in Christ's afflictions in behalf of His body, which is the church. I was made a minister of this church according to the commission from God granted to me for your benefit, so that I might fully carry out the preaching of the word of God, that is, the mystery which had been hidden from the past ages and generations, but now has been revealed to His saints, to whom God willed to make known what the wealth of the glory of this mystery among the Gentiles is, **the mystery that is Christ in you, the hope of glory.**

(Colossians 1:24–27)

There are some truths of God that are so massive, so expansive, and so all-encompassing that our minds boggle when we contemplate them. As a result, we don't think much on them at all.

Paul, on the other hand, didn't shy away from these mysterious truths. In fact, he sought to make them practical certainties. To the Thessalonians, he wrote:

May God himself, the God who makes everything holy and whole, make you holy and whole, put you together—spirit, soul, and body—and keep you fit for the coming of our Master, Jesus Christ. The One who called you is completely dependable. If he said it, he'll do it!

(1 Thessalonians 5:23–24 MSG)

Isn't that a thrilling thought? He who calls you is utterly faithful, and He will finish what He set out to do.

Paul is saying that the new creation that has begun in us is going to be finished—that is, if we allow it to be finished. Paul is praying for healing and wholeness. He is affirming the fact that every person, and Christians in a unique way, can find that inner harmony and peace.

Do not be surprised when people you know who have had a genuine conversion experience seek prayer because they are now plagued by fear and anxiety. They are devastated by recurring periods of depression. They find themselves still prone to physical maladies such as chronic headaches and ulcers, which are often rooted in emotional and spiritual causes.

They are justified by faith—but they know that they are not yet well.

They stay tired and weary because they spend their energy battling unresolved guilt or fighting off depression. We forget that the Christian experience is more than an intellectual profession of faith. Conversion— earnestly repenting of our sins and accepting Christ as Savior and Lord— is only the barest of beginnings in our Christian experience.

WE ARE NOT "ZAPPED INTO WHOLENESS." RATHER, WE GROW THROUGH "THE STEADY PRACTICE OF GODLINESS."

Paul pleaded with the Philippians to *"work out your own salvation with fear and trembling"* (Philippians 2:12). These people were already converted and profoundly Christian. This was Paul's favorite church, the one that supported him when no one else did.

So then, what does *working out our salvation* mean? Salvation certainly means receiving the grace of having our sins forgiven, yet it means far more. The word *salvation* comes from the same Latin root as the word *salve,* an ointment for healing. For this reason, Paul could only pray that the God of peace would make us "whol-ly"—that is, whole through and through. (See 1 Thessalonians 5:23.) His goal was that we would be kept in spotless integrity. The meaning of integrity is wholeness, the state of being complete and undivided.

As those who are learning to pray, we need to cultivate our personal awareness of the indwelling Christ as a healing and forgiving Presence. We need to pray with the confidence that Christ truly does offer healing and forgiveness to those for whom we pray.

In my (Maxie's) *Workbook on Becoming Alive in Christ,* I shared a personal experience that vividly connects our life *in Christ* and dimensions of healing prayer.

While I was preaching some special evangelistic services, I kept seeing a certain young man every day—in the morning and in the evening. I was introduced to him, and I could tell that something was going on in his life.

His eyes were troubled and searching; there was a tightness about his face that betrayed a troubled spirit.

Finally, he got up the nerve to ask to see me.

He came to my motel in the afternoon and began to share his story. He told me about his past life of sexual promiscuity and an abortion on the part of the one he loved but to whom he was not then married. Then he spoke of their marriage and their life together.

They now had one child and were a happy family. Yet he was stricken with ravaging guilt that was accentuating his physical illness, rooted in remorse over his past sin.

He felt himself to be a failure in his life in so many ways. But now, added to his guilt, was that haunting feeling, that ravaging, tearing-apart feeling, that his present illness was actually a form of God's punishment for his past sins.

He thought *God* had intentionally made him sick because he had sinned!

I shared the gospel as clearly as I could and talked about God's forgiving grace, the love of Jesus, and God's call to repentance. The young man received the gospel, repented, and was reborn as clearly as anyone I know could be reborn. He went rejoicing from our time together. I kept in touch with him for about a year after, and it was clear that his repentance was genuine and forgiveness had saved him from the ravages of guilt.

That's a dramatic story, and it doesn't always happen that way. But there are enough of these dramatic stories to keep getting our attention, to keep reminding us that Jesus calls us to repentance, a complete turning away from any known wrong. The gospel's offer is forgiveness and new birth, freedom from sin and wholeness of life. In one of Jesus's first healing miracles recorded in Mark's gospel, He connects forgiveness and healing.

A few days later, when Jesus again entered Capernaum, the people heard that he had come home. They gathered in such large numbers that there was no room left, not even outside the door, and he preached the word to them. Some men came, bringing to him a paralyzed man, carried by four of them. Since they could not get him to Jesus because of the crowd, they made an opening in the roof above Jesus by digging through it and then lowered the mat the man was lying on. When Jesus saw their faith, he said to the paralyzed man, "Son, your sins are forgiven." Now some teachers of the law were sitting there, thinking to themselves, "Why does this fellow talk like that? He's blaspheming! Who can forgive sins but God alone?" Immediately Jesus knew in his spirit that this was what they were thinking in their hearts, and he said to them, "Why are you thinking these things? Which is easier: to say to this paralyzed man, 'Your sins are forgiven,' or to say, 'Get up, take your mat and walk'? But I want you to know that the Son of Man has authority on earth to forgive sins." So he said to the man, "I tell you, get up, take your mat and go home." He got up, took his mat and walked out in full view of them all. This amazed everyone and they praised God, saying, "We have never seen anything like this!"

(Mark 2:1–12 NIV)

Here, Jesus makes it clear that there can be an intimate link between forgiveness and healing. Let's slow down and examine this text to understand this important connection, in the mind of Jesus—and then the crowd, the disciples, the early church, and Mark, who wrote the gospel.

The paralytic is at once pathetic and hopeful, both tragic and heroic. He is a "victim," carried about on a stretcher, yet he has courageous and hopeful friends who won't cease believing that there is help. They are bold in their pursuit of healing—tearing a hole in the ceiling of the house where Jesus is teaching in order to get their sick companion into Christ's Presence.

Two astounding dynamics are present:

1. The faith of the man and the four fellows who brought him

2. Jesus's immediate but puzzling response: "Son, your sins are forgiven"

The man's friends must have thought, *What's going on here? Our friend can't walk; we want him up and out of the stretcher. We have not even thought about sin and forgiveness.* They must also have been as deeply puzzled as others in the crowd. Likely they were shocked at Jesus's immediate word to the man and surprised by Jesus asking, "*Which is easier: to say to this paralyzed man, 'Your sins are forgiven,' or to say, 'Get up, take your mat and walk'?*"

Mark records that Jesus explained His reason for doing this.

Some in that crowd were balking at the implication that Jesus could forgive sins. This led to the dramatic moment named in the text—the question about what was easier to do, say a few words or perform a miraculous healing. *Clearly this healing was linked to the man's conscious memory of being sinful and unworthy.*

We know the end of the story. The fellow sprang to his feet, picked up his bed and walked away, leaving no doubt about the power of Jesus to heal and forgive.

In chapter 12, we will warn against *believing that sickness is always a consequence of someone's sin.* It is an open question whether Jesus connected physical and spiritual disease in a direct, regular, cause-and-effect fashion. Yet there is no room to doubt that Jesus connected tangibly experienced forgiveness and physical healing! He also made it clear that there is a connection between our spiritual health and our physical and mental well-being. For that reason, as intercessors, we should stay aware of the indwelling Christ as a healing Presence.

AS WE ABIDE IN CHRIST, A MAGNIFICENT DYNAMIC BECOMES ORDINARY. OUR PRAYER BECOMES OUR LIFE; OUR LIFE BECOMES OUR PRAYER.

It is what we mean when we talk about *an intercessory life.* This is a breathtaking truth. We become one with Christ, thus becoming "little Christs." C. S. Lewis expressed it boldly:

The church exists for nothing else but to draw men into Christ, to make them little Christs. If they are not doing that, all the cathedrals, clergy, missions, sermons, even the Bible itself, are simply a waste of time. God became man for no other purpose. It is doubtful...whether the whole universe was created for any other purpose. It says in the Bible that the whole universe was made for Christ and that everything is to be gathered together in him.[23]

Most writers on prayer, in all its practices, speak about intercession as a form of prayer. It most certainly is, yet it is more.

> *LIVING PRAYER IS THE LIFESTYLE OF CHRIST FOLLOWERS. WE LIVE INTERCESSORY LIVES.*

There will be more on this in chapter 11. We insist that we deliberately place ourselves in the company of the Holy Spirit, asking God to cleanse us of anything that separates us from *union with Christ*. We deliberately invite the Holy Spirit to join us to the power, grace, and holiness of the risen Christ. In this way, we are actually praying with our Lord Christ whose ministry is described in Hebrews:

> *Therefore he is able to save completely those who come to God through him, because he always lives to intercede for them.*
>
> (Hebrews 7:25 NIV)

Throughout this book, we have (and will) present Bible narratives of Jesus's power to heal, along with testimonies of those who have prayed or received healing prayer. The reason we have provided so many witnesses and described so many healings is not to answer all of the questions and mystery that will persist. We have sought to present credible testimonies, and the clear witness of Scripture, that Christ is the Healer and our praying is in partnership with Him.

We have built our theology of prayer for healing around the incredible truth that Jesus *"always lives to intercede"* (Hebrews 7:25 NIV).

He is praying for me. He is praying for you, even now, and He always will.

---

23. C. S. Lewis, *Mere Christianity*, quoted by Richard J. Foster, *Devotional Classics* (New York: HarperCollins, 1993), 10.

REFLECT AND RECORD

1. Maxie makes a strong case for two principles to be at work in every life: justification (getting saved) and abiding (letting Christ's Presence within you guide every action). Read what he says about the second and note what this means to you:

   The Presence of God in Jesus Christ is not to be experienced only on occasion; rather, the indwelling Christ is to become the shaping power of our lives.

   _____

   _____

   _____

2. This quote is stated in slang to capture a profound truth:

   We are not "zapped into wholeness." Rather, we grow through "the steady practice of godliness."

   This would be a paraphrase of this text, which tells us to *"work out your own salvation with fear and trembling"* (Philippians 2:12). Are you tempted to shortchange the need for steady disciplines to grow in grace? What steps do you practice to grow in godliness?

   _____

   _____

   _____

3. Reread Mark 2:1–12. Clearly healing and the acceptance of being forgiven are intertwined in this account of the paralytic. What does this say about emotional and physical healing?

   _____

   _____

   _____

A PRAYER FOR A LIFE CENTERED ON THE INDWELLING CHRIST

O God, there is beauty in this affirmation: "Our prayer becomes our life; our life becomes our prayer." Teach me to be so aware of the indwelling Christ in all I do that praying becomes like breathing—something that I do without preplanning or focused thinking. Make my life a prayer to You, all day, every day. Grant that I become one of those "little Christs." Amen.

8

HEALING: PRAYING, TOUCHING, SPEAKING

In the last chapter, we quoted C. S. Lewis saying boldly, *"The church exists for nothing else but to draw men into Christ, to make them little Christs."*

We used this expression from Lewis's writing to make the claim that our intercession is more than praying words. We are called to live intercessory lives. In this chapter, we want to discuss healing that involves more than our *praying words*, though that is primary to our theme. We believe that *touching* and *speaking* can be acts of prayer that bring healing as well. Our praying experiences often give us the opportunity to speak and touch in ways that heal or add to the healing experience.

Though we know that Lewis's claim that we are called to be "little Christs" is tough to grapple with, we want to continue that discussion with what may be a tougher claim, straight from the apostle Paul: *"Therefore be imitators of God"* (Ephesians 5:1).

That is an astounding command.

None of us can manufacture stars, commission angels to perform their tasks, order the affairs of eight billion souls at once, or even do as the risen Lord did by showing up disguised to two people on a road, vanishing from their sight, then materializing in another room just while those two are talking about us, only to eat a piece of fish. (See Luke 24:1–43.)

We might just manage to eat the fish—the rest would be out of bounds!

How then can we imitate God?

To get at that answer, we need to put the command within its proper context, both the previous verse, just before this bold command, and the one that follows. Taken together they show us how to be *"imitators of God."*

> **Be kind to one another, compassionate, forgiving each other,** *just as God in Christ also has forgiven you. Therefore be imitators of God, as beloved children; and walk in love, just as Christ also loved you and gave Himself up for us, an offering and a sacrifice to God as a fragrant aroma.* (Ephesians 4:32–5:2)

PRACTICE KINDNESS AND RECIPROCAL FORGIVENESS. BE FORGIVEN AND FORGIVE. THIS IS HOW WE ARE COMMANDED TO IMITATE GOD IN CHRIST.

Paul's writing helps us again with his word to another church—a young and immature assembly that needed his wise counsel after they more than slighted him. In fact, they hurt him, treated him poorly, didn't pay him a dime, called him a substandard preacher, and threw out some foundational and basic teachings of the faith, like the cross and the resurrection! In our minds, we would find it difficult to conceive of them as Christian at all!

Yet Paul thanked God for them!

This church was likely no more than three or four years in the faith, having been converted out of abject pagan idolatry. They were the Corinthians. Paul had already modeled gentle kindness and restraint in his first letter to them (although we can feel his hurt in 1 Corinthians 4:8–13). Somehow the apostle taught them of selfless love in chapter 13 of his first letter—and now in the second, the apostle teaches gentle kindness and restraint to them:

So from now on we regard no one from a worldly point of view. Though we once regarded Christ in this way, we do so no longer. Therefore, if anyone is in Christ, the new creation has come: The old has gone, the new is here! **All this is from God, who reconciled us to himself through Christ and gave us the ministry of reconciliation:** *that God was reconciling the world to himself in Christ, not counting people's sins against them. And he has committed to us the message of reconciliation.*
(2 Corinthians 5:16–19 NIV)

Paul names the one dynamic Christians are to keep alive: *"All this is from God, who reconciled us to himself through Christ and gave us the ministry of reconciliation"* (verse 18).

Reconciliation is the ministry to which we are called.

Ephesians 4:30–5:2 tells us to *"imitate God"* by forgiving, just as God in Christ forgave us.

Second Corinthians 5 tells us that the dynamic of reconciliation is forgiveness. Saying "yes" to forgiveness is saying "yes" to God's call.

In his word to the Corinthians, Paul was talking about *the practice of having God's perspective*—not viewing persons from a human point of view, but from heaven's. And when we have that perspective, the ministry of reconciliation follows.

On June 17, 2015, in Charleston, South Carolina, a white man, Dylann Storm Roof, murdered nine members of Mother Emanuel African Methodist Episcopal Church, including its lead pastor Clementa C. Pinckney, who was also a state senator. If members of that church or any other group had sought revenge, it might well have triggered a race war. Instead, the victims' families decided to forgive Dylann Roof. The act of forgiveness was so powerful that within two months, the Confederate flag was removed from the statehouse grounds in Columbia, South Carolina. An unforgettable message of reconciliation was sent across the world.

The families of the nine people who were killed and members of the Mother Emanuel AME Church practiced a core expression of the Christian faith. In fact, the apostle Paul said reconciliation is the ministry to which we are all called. After affirming the new life that is ours, he said, *"All this is from God, who through Christ reconciled us to himself and gave us the ministry of reconciliation"* (2 Corinthians 5:18 ESV).

Let's come at this in a slightly different way.

When are we most like God? We are most like God when we are most like Christ. And when are we most like Christ? We find our answer in Paul's word immediately preceding the Scripture we have been considering:

> *For Christ's love compels us, because we are convinced that one died for all, and therefore all died. And he died for all, that those who live should no longer live for themselves but for him who died for them and was raised again.* (2 Corinthians 5:14–15 NIV)

What an encompassing statement! *"We are convinced that (Christ) died for all."* Since He *has* died for all, He has died for each of us, and that is the great solvent by which the love of God melts our hearts and heals our fallen world.

HEALING BY SPEAKING

Sometimes our words are the healing dynamic of that love.

I (Maxie) have a friend, Mary Levack, a former Roman Catholic nun who entered a convent when she was young. Two sisters had done so before her. Mary told me her story late one night over coffee after I preached in the Methodist church where she was then serving in ministry as a lay person.

Mary's father left her mother with fourteen children when Mary was only five years old. You can imagine what that would do to a little girl—feeling abandoned, unloved, and unwanted. I was so moved, I asked her to record her testimony. Here is a part of that moving witness that verifies the claim that the love of Christ for each and for all is powerful, and sometimes, words are the healing dynamic:

> I entered the convent for two reasons. One, I felt the Lord calling me to a closer life with Him; and two, I was such a scrupulous individual and needed direction in the depths of my spirit because I did not really understand what this closer walk with the Lord meant for me; I was of the mind that I had to make up for my sins.

And so, as a teenager in the middle fifties, feeling it was time to do something with my life, I was of the opinion that it would be difficult for me to love one person to the exclusion of all others, and marriage therefore seemed out of the question even though I felt that was a stronger personal desire than going into the convent. But I needed to make up for my sins, and so, I thought God must be calling me into the convent.

Having been let into the convent, I was blessed. I found the Lord in a most beautifully intimate way. But I also found community life, and it was very threatening...Five years later, I ran away because it was too difficult for me in the sense that I was in too much inner turmoil. I wasn't a person who shared what was going on inside; I didn't know you could do that and be respected for it. So, I left the convent.

Because I hadn't been counseled properly, I went right into another depression and thought, Well, God, now I've really blown it—I've divorced the Lord, and I'm never going to get to heaven. So, I went back into my wounded position and cried and wept and prayed. Then I felt that God moved heaven and earth and even Rome as I was finally accepted back into the convent. Again, I was blessed. This time, I had a little more help in finding out what was really the source of the problem.

The word of the Lord came to me through a priest to whom I had admitted having entered the convent, among other reasons, for the sake of making up for my sins. When he heard this, he literally wept. And then he said, "Oh, my God, didn't anyone ever tell you Jesus did that. You don't have to do that. You can't do that. Just receive His forgiveness."

Well, at that time I was almost thirty years old, and I had just heard the good news, and praise God, it was from a Catholic priest.

Mary was healed, freed from a dark world of doubt and struggle, through the words she heard spoken aloud to her in a moment of crisis. Now she was serving as a lay minister in her church.

When are we most like Christ?

We are most like Christ when we are doing what He did in His extravagant gift of love on Calvary—forgiving. To speak that word can be a healing experience. Saying "yes" to forgiveness is our clearest witness to the fact that we are Christian.

In an upcoming chapter, we will suggest that a time of personal prayer is essential before we enter a time of praying for others. It is not likely that we will be able to pray earnestly for another to receive forgiveness when we need forgiveness ourselves.

We need to speak the word to ourselves: *"Christ has forgiven me!"*

Then we will be able to speak it with clarity and conviction to another: *"In the name of Christ, you are forgiven!"*

HEALING THROUGH TOUCH

In a number of ways and in many places in this book, we have underscored the healing power of touch. The call to lay *hands on* the person for whom we are praying is not accidental.

In the fifth chapter of Mark's gospel, there are three stories of healing. We examine parts of this chapter throughout *Healing Prayer*, especially in the "Reflect and Record" section at the end of chapter 6. What is worthy of consideration for our purposes here is that two of those healings involved *touching*.

Jesus and His disciples had been going from town to town, preaching the gospel and healing people. Large crowds were clamoring to see and hear Jesus. One day, a man named Jairus, a synagogue official, came looking for Jesus. He fell down at the Lord's feet and begged Him to come to his house because his only daughter was gravely ill and dying. Jesus agreed to go with him and as they went, people began to press in around Jesus, *"pushing and jostling him"* (Mark 5:24 MSG). The people were so excited to be near Christ that they were pushing, shoving, and crowding in close to Him.

As we have seen in a previous chapter, in the crowd was a woman who had been hemorrhaging for twelve years. She had tried everything she knew to try, but had no relief, and no one had been able to cure her. She slipped up behind Jesus, working her way through the crowd… and when no one seemed to be looking, she reached out tentatively, fearfully, and touched the hem of His robe.

At once, for the first time in twelve years, the flow of blood stopped.

Jesus simultaneously *felt* or *sensed* that something special had happened; it was a unique touch, and He felt *power* or *strength* go out of Him. Immediately, He stopped, turned around, and asked, *"Who touched me?"* (Luke 8:45 MSG). The disciples were astonished by the question in the midst of all of the pushing, shoving, and jostling.

> *His disciples said, "What are you talking about? With this crowd pushing and jostling you, you're asking, 'Who touched me?' Dozens have touched you!"*   (Mark 5:31 MSG)

They couldn't tell a *push* from a *touch*.

Jesus could! He knew the difference and knew that it was a tender touch that had drawn strength out of Him. The woman had not expected that she would be detected, but when Jesus turned and asked that question, she knew that He knew, and she came forward trembling. She fell at His feet and confessed that she was the one who had touched the hem of His garment. In a rush of words, she explained why she had touched Him and how she had been instantly cured. Graciously, Jesus said to her, *"Daughter, your faith has made you well; go in peace"* (Mark 5:34).

The rest of the story is even more remarkable. Remember, Jesus is on His way to heal Jairus's daughter. "It was too late," they told him; she had already died!

We're sure at that moment, Jairus was devastated. His only daughter had been snatched away. But again, Jesus, aware of the power upon Him, was gracious, generous, and loving. We can imagine Him touching Jairus's shoulder when He said, *"Do not be afraid any longer; only believe, and she will be made well"* (Luke 8:50).

They went on to the house. The people were weeping and mourning. But Jesus went into the room where the little girl lay. We can easily imagine Him gently cradling her face in His hands.

Yet Mark's gospel does tell us exactly what happened in that room.

He did touch her, even though she had passed. She was dead and lying on her bed.

Taking the child by the hand, He said to her, "Talitha, kum!" (which translated means, "Little girl, I say to you, get up!") And immediately the girl got up and began to walk, for she was twelve years old. And immediately they were completely astonished. (Mark 5:41–42)

He took the dead girl's hand in His—and then He spoke.

The text indicates healing touch and a healing word—both touch and word together. He loved her into life, through touch and word, and then, so matter-of-factly, He told them to give her something to eat. (See Mark 5:43.)

In imitation of Christ, I (Maxie) have found it helpful to touch and speak the word of forgiveness. If I have prayed personally or with a group for a person who has expressed confession and repentance, I invite that person to face me and give me their hands; touch is an expression of intimacy and identification. Then I invite them to look me in the eye as I say directly to them, "In the name of Christ, you are forgiven."

If we believe in the priesthood of all believers, any Christian can take the authority to pray, touch, and speak that word. David and Elizabeth bring all three together in this testimony from their ministry.

TAMMY'S HEALING

My wife and I (David, Elizabeth, and twelve others) prayed with a young mom with a severe eye injury. While we were praying, a significant thing took place that changed her life and the lives of those who sought God on her behalf. But that is getting ahead of the story. This is how the events unfolded.

The account began when a grandmother from the church called the office to ask if a pastor could come over to pray for her granddaughter's child, who was quite ill and home from the hospital.

I took the call and found myself driving to the home of a young mom named Tammy who had four children, the youngest a babe in arms who wheezed as she breathed. The grandmother came along and introduced me to everyone in the room. After those introductions, Tammy allowed me to hold the baby. I was sitting in a comfortable chair and gently rocked her. With mom's permission, I tenderly placed my hand on the child's head and prayed for the little girl to recover.

She was asleep in a few minutes in a blissful, quiet kind of way. So I passed the sleeping infant back to her mom, and she settled down to cradle the little child in her arms. Grandma lingered as I went back to the church.

That Sunday, I gave an invitation to embrace the forgiveness of the Lord—and Tammy came forward to receive the gift of salvation. After a few months, as Tammy grew in faith, she wanted to help out at church, and she became a helper in the Sunday school.

Fast forward two months.

Cleaning up from a children's event one Thursday, Tammy was taking down some outdoor decorations. She pulled sharply on a piece of string attached to a thumbtack that was holding a decoration lodged in an outside window casing. It dislodged, and as Tammy yanked to take it down, the soiled tip of the thumbtack went straight toward her eyeball. It scratched, partially penetrated, and injured her eye. Tammy screamed with sudden pain; a neighbor heard her, dashed outside, and took her to the hospital. There, the doctor's initial assessment was that Tammy had lost 60 percent of her forward vision and 100 percent of her peripheral vision in that eye due to the injury.

That was more devastating than it would be to most of us. You see, Tammy was a single mom with four young children—and this would make for significant trouble.

Yet, even with this injury, significant pain, and an eye patch, after spending the wee hours of Thursday night and early Friday morning at the hospital, this young mom came to our Sunday school teachers' workshop the very next day—early Saturday morning. She was sitting in the hallway early, blanched with pain, a pain that was exacerbated whenever the patch on her eye allowed a bit of light to seep onto her wound. We saw her in obvious distress when we began to straggle in for the workshop.

She told us what had happened as we gathered about, concerned for her health.

Then it happened: While we were standing in that hallway, Barb, an elder's wife, looked at us and said, "We need to pray—God wants to heal Tammy!" Suddenly all of us in that hallway experienced what is called *the testimony of the Spirit*—five of us sensed and became aware of the same thing at the very same moment.

We *felt* an interior signal of increasing Presence. It was an indicator for us to enter into a time of healing prayer.

> THOSE OF US WHO PRAYED FELT RISING PEACE, COMPASSION FOR THE YOUNG MOM, INTERIOR FIRE, AND GROWING CONVICTION THAT WE MUST PRAY.

So we did.

Gathering in the seminar room, we asked whether we could place our hands on her. With her permission, we did; by now, there were fourteen of us. We gently began to ask the Lord to heal that wound.

Fiery Presence filled the praying as the fourteen of us asked God for her restoration. While we were praying, we asked Tammy what was happening inside her body.

"There is gentle warmth coming from five hands!" she said. She tapped my hand, my wife's hand, and those of three others in the room, including that elder's wife.

How can we describe this?

It was compassion, love for God, focused purpose, joined together with the conviction that this woman *must* be healed, combined with an astonishing awareness of God's Presence! Some would call this a *shared gift of faith*. My own view (David's) is that the gifts of healing were given to everyone in the room—all of those praying and the one receiving the healing. Regardless of what we call this experienced moment of faith, it caused most of us to gently weep as we prayed.

Prior to asking Tammy that question, she had been experiencing significant pain because of the light leaking through the edges of the eye patch. As we continued to pray, each one of us asking God to heal her, this began to gradually change. The throbbing ache arising from light shining on the tender wound began to diminish, even as we were interceding. Tammy began to relax as relief was granted. We kept praying, until all pain diminished and then vanished altogether. Then the sense of *God Presence* among us lifted. Her pulsing discomfort from leaking light and the full-on body pain from the injury were both gone.

Although Tammy was visibly relaxed and no longer in pain, we advised her to leave the patch on until she saw the eye doctor on Monday.

The doctor's jaw dropped open when he removed the patch two days after our healing prayer. After processing what he was seeing, he checked his medical notes from the emergency ward. Then he examined her eye again.

Then, to Tammy's (and his) great astonishment, he declared that there was absolutely nothing wrong with her eye!

Just to make sure, he did a series of tests and followed that with a standard eye examination. All the while, he was comparing his findings to the hospital files. After thorough testing, he declared that the eye had 20/20 vision straight ahead and 100 percent peripheral vision to the side.

Tammy was delighted, thankful to God, and blissfully relieved.

Our prayer team and the doctor were astonished.

And when Tammy testified in a church service a few weeks later, the entire congregation was in awe that God was still doing such things among His people.

What we didn't know was *the rest of the story.*

As she was testifying, I asked her what had brought her to church. Tammy told everyone that her praying grandmother never gave up on her, even when she didn't want to live for God. She pointed to her and told everyone there that her grandma always told her she loved her and that God loved her. This caused the entire church to sit up and pay attention.

"My child had been sent home, unresponsive to any medical treatment," Tammy said. "So I asked Grandma Mary if anyone would come and pray for my little girl. Pastor David, you came and prayed for my daughter, and as soon as you started to pray, the wheezing stopped. She fell asleep in your arms and woke up the next day completely well."

My jaw dropped.

Not only was I astounded, but so was the entire congregation. I had no idea. Neither did anyone else.

"When I saw that Jesus healed my little girl, I knew that I needed to commit my life to Christ and learn His ways. That was why I came to church that weekend. That is why I started to help in the Sunday school. And now, Jesus has healed my daughter and me, and I love the Lord."

There was not a dry eye in the house.

Jesus healed the little girl.

Jesus healed her mother.

Jesus healed the heart of a praying grandma who sought the Lord for almost twenty-five years, wanting Tammy to embrace the gospel.

Praying, touching, and speaking—all of these instruments of God's power were a part of that story.

REFLECT AND RECORD

1. The Bible commands us to imitate God. Here is the text that contains the command. Read it and take a moment to write down the behaviors needed for the imitation to be effective.

    Be kind to one another, compassionate, forgiving each other, just as God in Christ also has forgiven you. Therefore be imitators of God, as beloved children; and walk in love, just as Christ also loved you and gave Himself up for us, an offering and a sacrifice to God as a fragrant aroma. (Ephesians 4:32–5:2)

    To imitate God, I need to:

    a. _____

    b. _____

    c. _____

    d. _____

2. Maxie speaks of the power of touch and word together. To be agents of God's grace, we ask to gently touch those for whom we pray, even as we speak. Is this something that you can do to demonstrate God's care for another?

_____

_____

_____

3. Tammy's eye was beyond medical intervention—and God healed it. Then we discovered that Tammy's daughter's sickness was beyond medical intervention as well, and God healed her! Then we discovered that behind it all was a praying grandmother who sought the Lord for more than twenty years. What does this say to you about how God heals?

_____

_____

_____

A PRAYER OF CONSECRATION

Lord, we know that speaking truth can be powerful. You spoke, and the world came into existence. In the healing of Jairus's daughter, You touched her hand even as You spoke to her spirit to return. Grant that our words and our presence convey Your grace—every action, every touch, every word. Amen.

9

SO—DID JESUS PRAY THIS WAY?

DEEP INTERCESSION IS GOD'S SPIRIT PRAYING
THROUGH ALL THAT WE ARE.

To begin a conference or a weekend event, it is always wise to start with a bit of fun just to help people relax and start to focus. One of my (David's) favorite teaser things to do is to ask this simple question:

"What is the shortest verse in the Bible?"

The responses are usually immediate. Either a cluster of hands shoot up straightaway to get my attention, or someone shouts out the answer: *"Jesus wept,"* they say with great gusto, quoting John 11:35. Sometimes the whole congregation says it together! If that happens, we all laugh a bit, and I hold up a prize—usually one of my books. Then I say, "If you want to win the prize, tell me the *second* shortest verse in the Bible."

The crowd looks blankly about until someone starts to laugh. The local Bible memorization aficionado or sometimes a child will say, *"Rejoice always!"* from 1 Thessalonians 5:16, or perhaps the next verse after it, *"Pray continually"* (NIV). Every now and then someone says, *"Remember Lot's wife!"* from Luke 17:32. And of course, the congregation laughs again, and some *Scripture memory hero* comes up to the front to get the prize. I ask the congregation to give the person a round of applause, and we laugh again! In this way, the ice is broken. Anyone who named 1 Thessalonians 5:16 or 5:17 or even Luke 17:32 wins the book.

Now, this gentle teasing bit of fun points to something that few have attempted to answer regarding that shortest verse.

Why did Jesus of Nazareth weep?

The answers to that question are many—usually pertaining to profound love, sympathy, or grief. The context, of course, was the death and burial of a close friend, Lazarus, and the grief of his two sisters, Mary and Martha. Neither sister could understand why Jesus didn't leave everything to race toward the dying man, to heal him, as He had healed so very many before under their watchful gaze. They lamented that He didn't head their way when the messengers had told Jesus that Lazarus was very ill. In fact, even the crowd shared in that lament:

> *But some of them said, "Could not he who opened the eyes of the blind man have kept this man from dying?"*   (John 11:37 NIV)

Martha said as much to Him. (See verse 21.) So did Mary, as she groaned with tears of grief. (See verse 32.)

In fact, Jesus Himself had told the disciples that Lazarus's illness would not lead to death! Most inconveniently, Lazarus died—and here is that same Jesus, traveling together with the twelve men He told, *"This sickness will not end in death"* (John 11:4 NIV), visiting *after* the man was not only dead, but had been dead and *"in the tomb for four days"* (John 11:17 NIV).

That meant that he was dead for five or even six days by the time Jesus got there.

Yet there is a corollary to this scene.

Two days *after* the Lord had said that His friend's sickness would not end in death (verse 4), He had told the disciples in plain speech that Lazarus had died, and that He was going to raise the man from the tomb. (See John 11:11–14.)

Follow the rest of the narrative, and we know the end of the story—Jesus visited the family and then the tomb, had the stone removed (despite a warning about the stench), shouted out for Lazarus to be raised—and the dead man lived. He rose despite being covered in binding cloth with seventy-five pounds of spices in a closed tomb in the Middle Eastern heat for four days.

We know from the beginning of John 11 that Jesus knew He would raise the man from death itself. So…

Why did Jesus weep?

JESUS WAS INVOLVED IN A DAYS-LONG INTERCESSION THAT INCLUDED HIM RECEIVING HIS ASSIGNMENT FROM THE FATHER BEFORE THE MESSENGERS ARRIVED.

The whole process was complex and growing. Jesus was given a cognitive download about His task, a waiting on God's timing, travel on foot, groaning tears, weeping, and deep emotion from every part of His earthly body. Finally, along with the two sisters, He had to exercise faith by having the stone removed and then shout at the top of His lungs, **"Lazarus, come out!"** (John 11:43).

Did you notice the in-depth involvement of the earthly Lord in this intercession? All of Jesus's physical, mental, emotional, and spiritual resources were focused on this prayer for resurrection. He was assigned to pray this way, and He did. The intercession ended when Jesus shouted, and Lazarus was raised.

Why did Jesus weep?

Jesus wept because He was engaged in a prayer process that covered the better part of a week; it was a growing, expanding prayer, a deep intercession. In fact, we are told by the writer of Hebrews that the regular practice of Jesus's prayer life included this very thing.

> *During the days of Jesus' life on earth, he offered up prayers and peti-*
> *tions with fervent cries and tears to the one who could save him from*
> *death, and he was heard because of his reverent submission.*
>
> (Hebrews 5:7 NIV)

Jesus's regular, consistent prayer practice included what some move-ments in church history have called *groaning intercession* or *the prayer of tears*. Most people who have been called to prayer like this know devotion-ally that this kind of praying is from God—yet they are afraid to name that it has happened to them as it seems so very unusual. In fact, we call it *whole-body intercession*.

It is defined by the apostle Paul in Romans 8. We mentioned this material in chapter 3 to quickly refer to the intercessor and the Lord's Spirit sharing their praying. In that chapter, Paul describes the creation being bought back from its slavery to corruption and death, climaxing in a prayer motif in which the Spirit and believers *pray together*.

1. The narrative begins with believers receiving Jesus's Spirit. It is called **"the Spirit of adoption as sons"** (Romans 8:15 ESV)—in which God's Spirit *speaks* or *testifies* and intertwines the Spirit of His Son, Jesus, with our human spirits—and we cry out, *"Abba! Father!"*—Christ has saved us! We become those characterized by the Spirit of Jesus the Son, resulting in our sharing in Jesus's relationship with God Almighty. (See Romans 8:14–17.) This leads to our assignment—the buying back of fallen earth through intercession.

2. Creation itself groans as those who are filled with the Spirit of God the Son walk upon its soil—eagerly yearning for the new and better day. (See Romans 8:18–22.)

3. Believers, filled with **"the first fruits of the Spirit"** (verse 23), groan inwardly as they wait for their resurrection bodies, yearning for that same better day when their new bodies are no longer inclined to sorrow, sin, and death. (See Romans 8:23–25.)

4. And the Spirit Himself groans, *praying through believers*—God's people, the church—as God Himself intercedes with Christ fol-lowers through their physical bodies via the indwelling Spirit.

God the Spirit now merges His praying with ours, as believers and God together pray to cause *"all things to work together for good to those who love God...[and] are called according to His purpose"* (Romans 8:28).

In this fourth point, it is clear that:

- ◆ Believers, who are infilled by the Spirit, and

- ◆ God, who is praying by His Spirit inside the believer

- ◆ Both together *feel their praying* at the same time.

They groan together in deep intercession as creation is reshaped by Jesus's Spirit (God's Presence) and Jesus's body (the church) praying in merged union together.

Do you see the theological point? God has shaped creation to respond to prayer offered by His children. So God joins His children to do this very thing! God enters into His predestined will that the world be transformed by the prayer ministry of the church.

Prayer is God's idea—to reshape the planet.

Healing prayer is God's idea to do the same!

> THE EARTHLY JESUS ENTERED INTO BOTH PRAYER AND HEALING PRAYER TO TRANSFORM US ALL TO BECOME JUST LIKE HIM! HE SENDS HIS SPIRIT TO PRAY THROUGH US TO DO JUST THAT!

To return to John 11, there are several moments in which it is clear that Jesus is praying *in the Spirit*. The late Gordon Fee would describe the intersection of the human spirit and the Holy Spirit by writing it in this manner, "Praying in S/spirit." Here, the Spirit of the Lord *testifies together* or *intertwines* with the spirit of the believer—the two witness or testify to each other—and deep intercession is born!

God's Spirit and the spirit of the intercessor groan together *"with groanings too deep for words"* (Romans 8:26). Intercessors, asking God to direct their praying, discover that God is *praying through them* by the intertwining of the Holy Spirit with theirs. They *feel* their praying, they groan together, and through that shared intercession, *"God causes all things to work together for good"* (verse 28). God's Spirit prays through us—and we feel it—to reshape the world through that deep intercession process. The least that can happen through this is that we become more like Christ.

> For whom He foreknew, He also predestined to be conformed to the image of His Son, that He might be the firstborn among many brethren. (Romans 8:29 NKJV)

With this understanding in our minds, let us reexamine John 11.

Jesus met Martha and spoke words of faith about the future resurrection. Then Mary sought Him out. Notice the language of the material as it relates to the inner spirit of Jesus:

> When Mary reached the place where Jesus was and saw him, she fell at his feet and said, "Lord, if you had been here, my brother would not have died." When Jesus saw her weeping, and the Jews who had come along with her also weeping, **he was deeply moved in spirit and troubled.** "Where have you laid him?" he asked. "Come and see, Lord," they replied. Jesus wept. (John 11:32–35 NIV)

Let's connect the dots.

Jesus was on His way to raise Lazarus from the dead—He had said it bluntly in John 11:11–14. He met the man's weeping sister and experienced an internal sensation of being *"deeply moved in spirit and troubled."*

It was right after this that *"Jesus wept."*

Yet the goal of the intercession had not yet been achieved. Lazarus was still lying dead in the tomb.

So Christ inquired about where the body was laid. In this next section, in His thanksgiving before the resurrection event, it becomes clear that Jesus had been praying this entire time about the matter. Here, *Christ was moved internally a second time*, and He thanks God that the prayer was accomplished—even before the answer is granted. To make it clear that this was a prayer event, we've highlighted the language about Jesus's inner being and His prayer before the miracle:

> Jesus, **once more deeply moved**, came to the tomb. It was a cave with a stone laid across the entrance. "Take away the stone," he said. "But, Lord," said Martha, the sister of the dead man, "by this time there is a bad odor, for he has been there four days." Then Jesus said, "Did I not tell you that if you believe, you will see the glory of God?" So they took away the stone. Then Jesus looked up and said, "**Father, I thank you that you have heard me**. I knew that you always hear me, but I said this for the benefit of the people standing here, that they may believe that you sent me." When he had said this, Jesus called in a loud voice, "Lazarus, come out!" The dead man came out, his hands and feet wrapped with strips of linen, and a cloth around his face.
>
> (John 11:38–44 NIV)

Jesus wept because His entire being was caught up in deep intercession concerning a resurrection event. His thanksgiving focused on the fact that His prior praying was heard and answered, even before His bold declaration for the dead man to come out of the tomb.

JESUS PRAYED WITH HIS ENTIRE BODY, AS THE SPIRIT PRAYED THROUGH HIM.

In fact, He didn't mutter or whisper when He spoke to the dead man. He shouted!

Why did Jesus shout?

It was because that is what it would take: His whole being was engaged in the declaration, as are the bodies of many praying saints when they pray in the secret place. Our Lord wept as a direct result of being moved in S/spirit during His intercession for the raising of the dead man, Lazarus.

So did Paul the apostle, describing this process as the means by which God *"causes all things to work together for good"* (Romans 8:28).

So can we when the Spirit of God intersects with ours and births an intercession that requires focus, dedicated time, and endurance in the praying.

Jesus wept. It's likely that you will too when you are involved in deep intercession.

REFLECT AND RECORD

1. A common way of expressing grief is to say that we have been *moved to tears*. Here, Jesus has that very thing happen to Him in His entire body. Have you ever been *moved* in your whole body when you have prayed? Describe this.

   _____

   _____

   _____

2. The apostle Paul describes *praying in and with the Spirit* as God's Spirit praying through us with groanings. What does this say about the value of prayer in God's sight? What does it say about how much God values those who pray?

   _____

   _____

   _____

3. Jesus groaned, wept loudly, and sometimes shouted when He prayed. What does this mean for us in times of praying?

   _____

   _____

   _____

4. There are other places in which we see this kind of groaning intercession in Jesus's ministry. Read the following Scripture from
Mark's gospel and ask yourself, "Did Jesus pray with His entire
body in this section?" After reading the text, record the things that
indicate that Jesus did in fact intercede with His whole being in
this healing prayer account:

> Then Jesus left the vicinity of Tyre and went through Sidon,
> down to the Sea of Galilee and into the region of the Decapolis.
> There some people brought to him a man who was deaf and
> could hardly talk, and they begged Jesus to place his hand on
> him. After he took him aside, away from the crowd, Jesus put
> his fingers into the man's ears. Then he spit and touched the
> man's tongue. He looked up to heaven and with a deep sigh said
> to him, "Ephphatha!" (which means "Be opened!"). At this, the
> man's ears were opened, his tongue was loosened and he began
> to speak plainly. (Mark 7:31–35 NIV)

What is the evidence from Mark 7 that Christ prayed not just with
His words but with His entire being?

_____

_____

_____

Notice that Jesus *sighed deeply*. The Greek word is often translated
"groaned." Was this a part of His praying? What does this mean
for our praying?

_____

_____

_____

A PRAYER OF SUBMISSION

Lord Jesus, You prayed with every part of who You are. We need to learn to do that too. I accept that Your Spirit can touch and flow through any part of who I am, even as He did within You during Your time on earth. Pray through me, as You will. Amen.

10

HOW WE PRAY FOR HEALING

As you approach an attitude of prayer, consider this:

Jesus is already interceding.

Isn't that a relief? You are simply joining in, like a child helping mom or dad with household chores. More important is this astonishing truth:

We are joining our imperfect prayers to His matchless ones.

We do not pray to someone far removed from us. The joy of the gospel is that we are *in Him* and He is *in us*. He knows us because He indwells us. We don't have to impress or convince God about anything. There is no need to prove ourselves to Him. Rather, we join our minds, hearts, and wills with those of Jesus, who is already interceding with the Father.

Remember, the Spirit of Christ already resides within you. Jesus's Spirit will stand with you as you attempt to begin to pray.

HOW WE PRAY

THE INNER POSTURE OF PRAYER

By God's design, we are partners with Christ in intercession!

Based on this, we pray *with* Christ, *through* Christ, and *in* Christ. Because prayer is God's idea, we begin with these attitudes as rock-solid footing, even before we start. We start praying by embracing these postures of faith:

- *Having bold confidence in going to God.* "Let us hold fast the confession of our hope without wavering, for he who promised is faithful" (Hebrews 10:23 ESV)

- *Trusting God's faithfulness.* "Faithful is He who calls you, and He also will do it" (1 Thessalonians 5:24)

- *With childlike simplicity.* "'Have faith in God,' Jesus answered. 'Truly I tell you, if anyone says to this mountain, 'Go, throw yourself into the sea,' and does not doubt in their heart but believes that what they say will happen, it will be done for them'" (Mark 11:22–23 NIV)

- *Confidently.* "Therefore, since we have a great high priest…Let us then approach God's throne of grace with confidence, so that we may receive mercy and find grace to help us in our time of need" (Hebrews 4:14, 16 NIV).

- *Remembering it is the Spirit who intercedes.* "In the same way the Spirit…intercedes for us with groanings too deep for words…He intercedes for the saints according to the will of God" (Romans 8:26–27).

- *Knowing Jesus esteems the desires of your heart.* "I chose you and appointed you so that you might go and bear fruit—fruit that will last—and so that whatever you ask in my name the Father will give you" (John 15:16 NIV)

As we grow in our walk with Christ, we find a simplicity in the way we dwell in God's Presence. Many faithful believers who came before us have written beautifully on the spiritual truths of our shared walk with God. Those who wrote down their wisdom often spoke of the certain joy of walking with God, even in the times of hardship or the ups and downs of everyday life. Praying over serious matters does not mean we take ourselves too seriously. Remember, Jesus was amazed and perhaps laughed with joy when He realized the faith of the centurion. (See Matthew 8:10.)

We can laugh too!

AS PATIENT LEARNERS

Jesus began His ministry through being filled with the Spirit's power at His baptism. That same Spirit then led Him into His first prayer assignment: He prayed and fasted for forty days in the wilderness against a backdrop of sharp temptation. To win back every level of what it means to be human, Jesus, the second Adam, filled with the Spirit, defeated the tempter's taunts physically, then mentally and emotionally, and finally spiritually—before commanding the devil to leave.

This time of prayer and testing was then followed by Christ beginning His ministry of preaching, healing, and saving.

No ministry happened until after:

+ Christ was filled with the Holy Spirit.

+ Jesus was commanded to pray for forty days.

+ Jesus defeated the enemy of our souls on all levels of what it means to be human.

After all that—and only after all that—Jesus got started!

Among the disciples who started to follow Him, however imperfectly, was Simon Peter. We are old friends with Simon! It gives us great joy to know that Jesus chose him to lead the church. Peter's story gives great hope to all of us!

Peter was warmly human, a seasoned outdoorsman, a fisherman who demonstrated a combination of good-heartedness, bluster, and an impulsive nature. Peter would step out and get it right, then almost immediately fall flat on his face again. Jesus kept inviting Peter back again, more than once, into deeper growth—and even repeated a miraculous catch of fish to call him back after his most catastrophic failure. (See Luke 5:1–11; John 21:1–19.) And this was *before* Pentecost, when the Holy Spirit fell on all of those gathered in prayer to empower them, even as Jesus had been empowered.

So if Jesus could use Peter, Jesus can use you and me!

Jesus's patience with him will be true of His patience with us as well as we respond to the Holy Spirit's calling us into healing prayer. Praying for healing doesn't mean that we won't still learn and grow gradually, as those early followers did, even as the Holy Spirit lands us in the middle of the unexpected.

GOD DOES NOT NEED EXPERTS! GOD NEEDS SERVANTS OPEN TO GIVING THEMSELVES IN PRAYER.

If you are open to giving yourself in prayer, you are just as qualified as Simon Peter!

PRAYING TOGETHER

There were seasons in which Jesus sent out His disciples in pairs to go ahead of Him to preach and pray for healing. One of the earliest accounts we have of this tells of their work in teams and anointing sick people with oil for healing.

> *And He summoned the twelve and began to send them out in pairs, and gave them authority over the unclean spirits…They went out and preached that people are to repent…and were anointing with oil many sick people and healing them.* (Mark 6:7, 12–13)

Jesus wasted no time in sending His disciples to pray for the afflicted and expected them to see results from their ministry of intercession.

But He did not send them out alone. Jesus ensured that they went out in teams; they were ordinary people, not even priests or religious scholars. He didn't tap the rising stars of the Sanhedrin. He sent fishermen and two kinds of people from the radical edges of His time: a tax collector (a collaborator with the invading empire) and a rebel zealot—an extremely unlikely partnership. Some teach that these two would have been avowed enemies under any other circumstances.[24]

---

24. It is possible that Simon the Zealot may have belonged to a group of nationalistic Jews who would resort to violence in the name of the faith of Israel. It is also possible that this name may refer to Simon being "characterized by zeal" for the Lord. Either way, that a tax collector should share company with those zealous for God's law is an unlikely, even volatile, combination under any circumstance.

Members of this motley crew were sent out in public together—not to fight or brawl, but to pray and heal.

On some matters, we pray on our own. Yet prayer for healing often occurs when groups of people gather or in a team of intercessors. In this way, individuals' particular and unique spiritual gifts and experiences are brought into the mix as the prayer begins. When someone faces a health crisis, an awful diagnosis, or simply a significant need, we need each other!

We need the church; a community of believers is essential in prayer for healing. Even Jesus didn't want to pray alone when He went to the garden of Gethsemane. He yearned for friendship and prayer partnership even then!

If God the Son needed companionship in prayer, how much more do the rest of us need that fellowship! Churches exist as communities of faith to speak to God together, praying for His intervention to spare a life or restore health and well-being.

In his epistle, James tells us we need each other to pray for healing. His words make it clear that the church he was writing to was anything but perfect! Yet these imperfect souls need each other when someone is ill.

> *Is anyone among you in trouble? Let them pray. Is anyone happy? Let them sing songs of praise. Is anyone among you sick? Let them call the elders of the church to pray over them and anoint them with oil in the name of the Lord. And the prayer offered in faith will make the sick person well; the Lord will raise them up. If they have sinned, they will be forgiven. Therefore confess your sins to each other and pray for each other so that you may be healed. The prayer of a righteous person is powerful and effective.* (James 5:13–16 NIV)

Note the different responses to different circumstances in life. In verse 13, *"in trouble"* refers to misfortune or difficulty in ordinary life. In this circumstance, the believer is encouraged to pray for God to intervene and transform trouble into relief. In the same verse, *"happy"* suggests someone who is in good spirits, joyfully encouraged, whose circumstances are going well. These believers are encouraged to practice singing out their praises to God, whether alone by themselves or together with others.

But for those who are *"sick"* in verse 14, there is a combination of being both weak and physically ill—the kind of illness that could almost render one helpless. Imagine someone very ill in intensive care, unable even to get up independently.

The thrust of the text is clear:

+   If we are ill, we should ask for help.

+   If we are well, we should be ready to go and pray for those who are sick.

This doesn't mean that you need to call the prayer team before an annual checkup or a root canal, but it does mean that followers of Christ acknowledge that ultimately, our bodies belong to God! Eventually, everyone will face something beyond their control or influence to change. Facing the limits of our own bodies—and recognizing that all of us are going to die—helps us see the moments when we should ask others for help and pray without fear.

Healing prayer often takes place through a team.

In James 5, it is clear that those being asked to pray were not the original twelve apostles, nor even a church pastor. Those who are asked to join in prayer for healing were believers whose walk with God had blossomed and grown in a local congregation. (At that time, believers met in house churches.) Their spiritual growth and maturity would have been clear to everyone who met in that house!

ASK THOSE WHOSE DEVOTION YOU TRUST TO PRAY FOR YOUR HEALTH.

In James's letter, those asked to pray had a solid walk with God, clearly demonstrated in their lives. They became *elders*. These are the ones to ask to pray for your healing.

One of the common marks of spiritual leadership is a developing, growing prayer life. Every church has people like this; they have *a sweet walk with God*, and they love people too!

Christian leaders have a prayer life that is ongoing and fruitful. They pray regardless of whether they have a formal role in the church.

YOUR PRAYER LIFE MAY RUN QUIETLY BUT DEEPLY. WHETHER YOU ARE INTROVERTED OR EXTRAVERTED, SHY OR OUTGOING, YOU CAN PRAY FOR OTHERS!

Together, believers are urged to pray in faith for the sick to be made well by God's powerful intervention. Praying for healing with others in a team prevents abuses and ensures accountability.

TESTIMONY: TRANSPARENCY AND VULNERABILITY

We know some of them, and maybe you do too. They look just like you and me. And that's the issue. Some church leaders have taken advantage of and hurt people. Worse yet, they hurt people under the guise of doing good in Jesus's name. Their actions ruined the good name of the church.

As heartbreaking stories of predatory leaders rock the church all across the earth, it is all the more urgent that we develop approaches that make praying with others safe and aboveboard.

Our approaches need to be transparent, respect the vulnerable, serve with sensitivity to trauma, and promote emotionally healthy ministry.[25]

Jesus condemned spiritual abuse in the strongest language:

If anyone causes one of these little ones—those who believe in me—to stumble, it would be better for them to have a large millstone hung around their neck and to be drowned in the depths of the sea. Woe to

---

25. See Diane Langberg, *Redeeming Power: Understanding Authority and Abuse in the Church* (Ada, MI: Brazos Press, 2020).

> *the world because of the things that cause people to stumble! Such things*
> *must come, but woe to the person through whom they come!*
>
> (Matthew 18:6–7 NIV)

Every person who prays for another has been given a gift from God. We are to steward those moments as though they belong to Him, not us!

Even as we learn and grow, there are ways we can carry out praying for others to remove hurdles instead of adding them. Any kind of leader— especially in an era marked by abuse of trust—enters these moments to pray with another with humility.

In our congregations (and in the world), we find people bearing significant wounds. There are those scarred by deprivation and poverty, those burned by bad teaching, and those who have endured all kinds of abuse.

As we learn to pray *for* others, praying *with* others prevents misunderstandings, provides insights, and creates accountability for everyone's feedback and reflection. Here is an example of that approach:

At one point in ministry, I (Maxie) saw the powerful deliverance that came when a community of Christ followers loved, cared unconditionally for, believed in, and prayed with and for a deeply troubled young woman. In this case, the work of intercession or *standing in the gap* worked powerfully in her life.

She had been locked into a way of thinking that sealed her into believing that she could never be healed or escape. The power of shame and guilt had been at work for a long time. Abused as a child, she broke from that cycle of violence as a teenager, but lived for many years with shame and depression, unable to free herself from the destructive memories of that cruel violation. She was under psychiatric care as well as pastoral care from congregational ministers.

Before I knew her background, I had noted that she always kept her distance from me. One day at a gathering, I walked up to her, put my hand on her shoulder, and greeted her. She reacted strongly, and though I didn't understand why, I realized that somehow, I'd frightened her.

She moved away as quickly as she could without a word.

After that, the minister who knew her arranged a meeting, and as the three of us met, I learned her story.

As chance would have it, I bore a slight resemblance to her abuser, so my presence triggered a traumatic flashback. She had only told this to her psychiatrist and her pastoral counselor. Even in what seemed to me to be the safety of that room, her pastoral counselor seated beside her, she struggled to share her story. Thankful for the gifts and insights of the mental health professionals tending to her, when I learned of the heartbreaking reality in her life, I began to pray for her in my personal prayer time. I also knew that there were other discreet intercessors praying for her emotional and psychological healing and release from the grip of deep trauma.

I never will forget an experience that took place about a month later.

In an evening worship service of celebration, praise, and healing prayer, after receiving Holy Communion, people were invited to come to the altar for specific prayer with ministers. There were pastors on both sides of the space, and people usually approached the minister nearest to them. On this night, the young woman was seated on the opposite side from me. When people were invited to prayer, she almost ran across the front of the church to kneel before me.

It was obvious that a power not her own was propelling her.

Before that night, she couldn't have gotten within five feet of me. Now, she reached out to take my hands, and she began to pray. Her own prayer that evening, rooted in the acceptance, love, and prayer of the community of faith surrounding her, cast out and *exorcised the spirits* of shame, guilt, and depression. The Holy Spirit's Presence began to bring healing to the effects of trauma, like her plaguing certainty of worthlessness.

The Holy Spirit, God's healing Presence, prevailed over the flashbacks and fallout that had ruled her life day in and day out. The Spirit prevailed because the love of Jesus Christ had been expressed through a whole community of faith—a team consisting of pastors, an able and understanding therapist, and a prayer group who faithfully cared for her.

It took all of us together.

We utilized the best tools of therapy, showing respect for her space and timing. And we communicated with transparency to each other to help support her to the place in which she could bring the wounds of the past into the gentle healing light of Christ.

HEALING HANDS

In healing prayer, *proximity* or *nearness* of some kind is found time and again throughout the New Testament. Not only did the touch of Christ bring healing, but besides the well-known story of the woman with the hemorrhage in Mark 5, the gospel writers record many accounts of crowds attempting to touch Jesus's clothing.

What is astonishing for the modern mind to fathom is that the healing power resting in and upon Him would flow through the very fabric of His clothing. Here is what happened after Christ spent the night in prayer and selected the Twelve:

> *Jesus came down with them and stood on a level place; and there was a large crowd of His disciples, and a great multitude of the people from all Judea and Jerusalem, and the coastal region of Tyre and Sidon, who had come to hear Him and to be healed of their diseases; and those who were troubled by unclean spirits were being cured. And all the people were trying to touch Him, because power was coming from Him and healing them all.* (Luke 6:17–19)

On a couple of occasions, someone would approach Jesus to request healing for another who was incapacitated somewhere else. In speaking with them, Jesus would proclaim that the ill person was made well. (See, for example, Luke 7:2–10; Matthew 15:21–28.)

Beyond the ministry of Jesus of Nazareth, in Acts 5, we have the astonishing record of how clusters of signs and wonders happened through the ministry of the first apostles:

> *And increasingly believers in the Lord, large numbers of men and women, were being added to their number, to such an extent that they even carried the sick out into the streets and laid them on cots and pallets, so that when Peter came by at least his shadow might fall on any of them. The people from the cities in the vicinity of Jerusalem were*

coming together as well, bringing people who were sick or tormented with unclean spirits, and they were all being healed.   (Acts 5:14–16)

Even the shadow of Simon Peter brought miraculous healing!

The New Testament speaks of many elements of healing prayer, including:

+ Touch and the laying on of hands

+ Physical nearness of an ill person or an advocate

+ A spoken request

+ Someone reaching out physically in an unspoken request for healing

+ Requests for prayers of healing spoken and prayed out loud

+ Touching a garment of Christ when He was anointed

All of these are included in the accounts of healing prayer in the Bible.

Through Jesus's Presence, the Holy Spirit's power would flow.

Invariably, a common feature in the healing accounts is that there was usually some form of physical contact. In one account, Jesus returned to a spot where He had healed ill people once before.

When they got out of the boat, immediately the people recognized Him, and ran about that entire country and began carrying here and there on their pallets those who were sick, to wherever they heard He was. And wherever He entered villages, or cities, or a countryside, they were laying the sick in the marketplaces and imploring Him that they might just touch the fringe of His cloak; and all who touched it were being healed. (Mark 6:54–56)

TESTIMONY: ANOINTING

Shortly after arriving at a particular congregation, I (David) was granted the privilege of performing a wedding ceremony for two retirees. When I met the bride to schedule preparations, our conversation landed on something remarkable. Susan shared that she had never thought she would see her wedding day because she had been diagnosed with a notoriously aggressive kind of pancreatic cancer and had been planning her funeral. She said she was told that on average, less than 10 percent of people with pancreatic cancer survive; if it has metastasized, the survival rate is close to zero.

Susan had received all of the medical treatments available to her, including chemotherapy and an invasive medical procedure that was her last best hope.

Then came the devastating news: the cancer had metastasized. It had spread into her lungs and other internal organs.

Even the specialists could do nothing. She was told that she might live three to six months under the best circumstances: three months was the timeline if she went untreated and perhaps as long as six months if she received aggressive chemotherapy.

Most diagnosed with this particular form of cancer die a rapid and painful death.

But for Susan, the outcome would be different.

She belonged to a small Bible study group, and she asked a couple of its members, who were elders from the congregation, if they would consider anointing her with oil to pray for her healing. She also asked several friends who were strong, faithful believers. And so they gathered together on Sunday, February 5, 2012—the day after World Cancer Day, which is held to raise awareness of this dreaded disease—to ask God for mercy.

The request was more than serious—it was life or death.

Everyone in the room loved Susan. They followed the leading they had, anointing her forehead with oil; then, at her invitation, everyone in the room gently placed their hands on her and began to pray.

As Susan told me the story of what happened during that remarkable prayer time, her eyes filled with tears. Her friends and two church elders had placed their hands on her to intercede before the Lord. Susan had trouble trying to put the experience into words. Her entire body had been filled with God's Presence.

I asked her to describe it.

She struggled for words and finally said it was "a combination of growing fiery heat" and "peace that passes understanding." That Presence gradually encompassed her entire body as she sensed within that God was actively healing her.

Suddenly, she simply "knew" it was done. Like the woman with the issue of blood, she "felt it in her body."

The prayer time was gentle, not demanding or pushy. God's Presence within turned into simple assurance that it was completed; she simply knew beyond knowing that God had done it.

Susan was healed.

I wish I had been there.

Yet a grace was given. Years later, I was granted the privilege of meeting several of those who were in the room during this healing prayer for Susan. I asked them to describe what they sensed as they prayed. Her friends remarked on the very same thing: as they began to pray for Susan, their bodies were filled with God's Presence, which felt like a combination of fire, peace, and joy. Two of her female friends were filled with complete conviction, a gift of extraordinary faith. They were utterly convinced that for God's glory, Susan must be made well! God's Presence filled them, then spilled over into their friend as they asked God to touch her body and remove the cancer.

One of the two elders testified that he sensed sudden filling as they all placed their hands on her shoulders. They were overwhelmed with an awareness of the majesty of God, brimming over with the love of Christ for their friend.

The elders, her three friends, and Susan herself all spoke of a shared experience as they placed their hands on her and prayed. They sensed "peace," "fiery warmth," "compassion," and a "holy conviction," a certain knowledge. They all suddenly knew that God was at work in her body, healing her of terminal cancer. Together, collectively, Susan and everyone else in the room received the overwhelming sense that the matter was done. She was healed.

When the prayer time ended, she was convinced that no further steps were needed, as modern medicine had reached its limit, and she believed she was well. Her intercessors encouraged her to continue cooperating with whatever the medical professionals might recommend. So although her physicians had told her it wouldn't do much good, she did in fact take chemotherapy, which in ordinary circumstances would only delay her inevitable death by a few months at the most.

She went in for a medical examination four months later.

Everyone except Susan was astonished to discover that there was not a trace of cancer in her body, and that she had gained some weight and had no body pain. Medically, this was impossible. Anyone who knows anything about cancer, especially pancreatic cancer, knows that metastasized cancer does not reverse. At the time of writing, that prayer time was nearly thirteen years ago, and Susan has had no trace of cancer to this day.

Everyone involved in that time of intercession for healing indicated that they felt God's Presence within them when they laid hands on her. This healing grace overflowing with the love of Christ was sensed internally. Susan felt healed within and received a *gift of faith*, knowing with simple certainty that God had acted.

HEALING BY SURPRISE

There is another dimension to be considered in the complex interactions of body, brain, spirit, memory, and mind. Occasionally, trauma is borne in the body, and healing emotionally, spiritually, and psychologically soothes the symptoms of the wounded body.

There is some speculation in emerging neuroscience that at times, the brain, overwhelmed by the pain of trauma, doesn't know where to process it, registering it as pain experienced in the body.

You can be heartsick and feel pain in your body.

Sometimes, undiagnosed chronic pain may be explained by simply recognizing that we have not yet learned about a particular disease. Care must be taken not to assume a psychological cause of physical symptoms.

For people who have thoroughly pursued every avenue medicine can offer and whose symptoms or pain continue, there are those unusual times in which healing prayer brings peace and healing to complex, trauma-driven physical symptoms.

God sees and cares for the whole person. As stated in chapter 7, Jesus spoke a word of forgiveness to a paralyzed man before He told him to take up his bed and walk. In this case, Jesus responded to the emotional and spiritual needs of the person in front of Him before telling him to rise and walk! (See Mark 2:1–12.)

SOMETIMES PHYSICAL HEALING BRINGS NEW HOPE, AND WITH IT, WE DISCOVER EMOTIONAL OR SOCIAL HEALING. SOMETIMES, EMOTIONAL OR PSYCHOLOGICAL HEALING BRINGS HEALING OF PHYSICAL SYMPTOMS.

Jean Watson, author of *Everything Can Change in Forty Days: A Journey of Transformation through Christ*, a symphony violinist, and an international speaker, was astonished to discover that God could use even her! She found, to her initial shock, God's healing grace at work in her praying. She notes, "Though I would never want to relive the years I suffered, I'm thankful to have walked that road. It was necessary to be completely broken so that God could use me for his glory and not mine."[26]

One day after giving a concert in Coventry, England, to an audience that included homeless people in a city ravaged by alcoholism, people responded to the Presence of the Holy Spirit and came forward for prayer, including a man and his twelve-year-old daughter.

Jean writes:

He explained she was losing her hearing and the doctors were baffled. Speaking on her behalf, he emphatically stated, "she believes that Jesus will heal her if you pray."

I remember thinking, *well, that's probably not going to happen, but people are watching. How can I refuse to prayer for her?* So, I

---

26. Jean Watson, *Everything Can Change in Forty Days: A Journey of Transformation through Christ* (Franklin, TN: Seedbed Publishing, 2018), 20–21.

placed my hands on the girl's ears and asked the Lord to touch her through me.

As I prayed, it felt like a million volts of electricity passed through us, causing me to fall backward and land on the floor. Astonished, I stood up and exclaimed, "Get away from me! I am a sinful woman. I am not worthy!" Later I remembered Peter had uttered something similar when he realized he was in the presence of Jesus the Christ (Luke 5:8).

At that moment there was such intense holiness around the girl that I knew she had been healed. Several weeks later her parents e-mailed me verification from the doctors showing that, indeed, her hearing had been restored. No one was more surprised by her healing than me. That night the Lord used a broken lady to shine his healing power into broken lives in a broken city. All he asked of me was to show up and be willing.[27]

But on a different night in a different city, Jean found herself witnessing the healing promise of God in a very different way, to a very different and complex person. She writes:

If we are willing, God may send us into some of the darkest places where his light is needed the most. The evening I arrived in Manchester some friends had planned an outreach event in the red-light district of the city. On that cold Friday evening, four of us drove into the heart of the city and asked for the Lord to reveal his love through us. As we prayed, I saw a face in my mind. She was a young woman with distinct features. I thought perhaps it was just my imagination, but I shared what I had seen with the others and asked God to bring this woman to us.[28]

As Jean and her team of friends drove around, they found an empty street corner and took hot drinks and sandwiches from the van, waiting for hungry women to emerge; they did. Then, Jean saw her—the woman whose features had come to mind in her prayer. She relates:

27. Ibid., 25–26.
28. Ibid., 109–110.

Unlike the others, she wore no makeup, and the side of her face was badly bruised. I was struck not by the bruises, but by the unmistakable beauty I saw underneath.

Without thinking, I yelled out, "You are *so* beautiful!"

This lady caught my eye and shouted back in lower-class urban British, "No, I'm not!"

I was able to come closer and explain how the Lord had brought me all the way from America to tell her. She begged me not to judge her. She showed me more bruises and an old stab wound on her leg. I explained that God loved her so much that he sent me halfway across the world just to tell her how beautiful she was.

I knew I couldn't convince [her] to believe in God's love. She would have to experience it for herself. I asked if I could pray with her, and she said yes.

Putting my arm around her shoulders, I prayed that the Lord would reveal his love to [her] in a way she could understand. After we prayed, she looked up with tears streaming down her face and said, "Don't stop touching me. God is in your hands!" I wondered if this was the first time [she] had ever been touched with love.[29]

Ministering with a team of other believers, Jean brought Jesus *near!* Through the close proximity of face-to-face interaction and her hands on the woman, by the power of the Holy Spirit, Jean brought God's loving Presence to a physically, emotionally, and spiritually bruised and wounded prostitute, who found herself unexpectedly experiencing the direct love of God in a supernatural, tangible way.

For Susan, the body of Christ gathered to anoint her with oil. They prayed as an act of love, with hands on her shoulders. The result was that the Holy Spirit's Presence filled her and those who were praying for her.

Touch.

Nearness.

Proximity.

The power of the Lord flowed through these means.

---

29. Ibid., 110–111.

As Jean relates, for one broken woman on a street corner, prayer, healing touch, and the supernatural gift of being unexpectedly seen all brought an abused prostitute face to face with the healing love of God for her—all of her, every dimension of her existence.

Jesus, the great Healer, desires all to welcome and receive the unmistakable love of God that brings hope, wholeness, and health.

REFLECT AND RECORD

1. In Susan's experience of healing, she received love from a caring fellowship of Christ followers in a medically impossible situation. Have you ever prayed for someone and sensed warmth or conviction that God was doing something beyond understanding? Have you ever been prayed for and experienced this?

_____

_____

_____

2. Jean Watson discovered *healing by surprise*—first in the unexpected physical healing of a young girl who simply asked her to pray, then how an emotional wound in a despairing, abused woman was healed through loving touch. What does this say about how God brings healing?

_____

_____

_____

3. Have you ever been on the receiving side of prayer and felt relief from some suffering, disease, or anxiety in your body? How would you describe it?

_____

_____

_____

A PRAYER FOR HEALING PRESENCE

Jesus, You became a human to fill every part of what it means to be human. Our bodies sometimes fail and break down. At other times, they are subjected to cruelty or trauma.

Yet one of the ways healing prayer goes to work is through human touch and love from others. You shine through our imperfections when we simply make ourselves available to You!

So, we offer You our bodies, our hands, our voices and words, our Presence, our time, and our availability; anoint us, we pray, and show us how to be a means not of harm but of Your love and transforming healing. Meet with us here and now, we pray.

Come, Holy Spirit. Amen.

11

PREPARING THEN PRAYING FOR HEALING

As the life of Christ illustrates so powerfully, an ongoing ministry of prayer for others, particularly prayer for healing, flows out of a close walk with God and spiritual friendship with other believers; it includes times of personal and gathered worship. Along with intentional spiritual growth in relationship with others, it is important to practice such things as being transparent and accountable. This makes for spiritual and emotional health.

The goal is to *build to last*, to shape a ministry that continues. Sustainable practices inside a community of faith allow each person and the team to thrive as they learn how to enter into God's idea—*healing prayer*.

To get ready for healing prayer, it is always wise to set apart time to pray on your own. Jesus practiced this. We have been in the ministry for a long time: David for more than thirty years and Maxie for more than sixty years. In every church we have served, the assumption was that if an area was growing, then we should do more of it!

Add another worship service!

Expand the Sunday school!

Do another outreach event!

Participate in another community project!

Grow—and get growing!

Usually that would have been the right thing to do. When the throngs were yearning for Jesus's teaching and ran around a lake just to be near to Christ, He did in fact accommodate their needs. He taught them and even fed them through miracles. (See Matthew 14:13–21, 15:32–38; Mark 6:33–44, 8:1–9; Luke 9:10–17; John 6:1–13.) Yet there was one singular exception to this:

IN JESUS'S MINISTRY, PRAYER IN THE PRIVATE, QUIET PLACE PRECEDED HEALING PRAYER IN PUBLIC.

A favorite passage to help in developing a theology of prayer has been Luke 5:12–15 in which Jesus healed a leper. It had this marvelous effect:

> *But the news about Him was spreading even farther, and large crowds were gathering to hear Him and to be healed of their sicknesses.*
>
> (Luke 5:15)

If that were us and our churches, we can both hear our excited voices and the joyful voices of our leaders saying, "Praise God! Many are being reached! The gospel is going forward! Let's add another service. It's clear that God's favor is on this. It is always wise to strike when the iron is hot."

In Luke 12:1, we are given some hard numbers and a vivid picture about the effect of Jesus's ministry: "*So many thousands of people had gathered together that they were stepping on one another.*"

What would your response to that kind of *crowd energy* be? We suspect that if you are anything like us, you would have wanted to add more opportunities to pray for the sick as well. The attitude is often, "If it is growing, add on!"

This is in stark contrast to the practice of Jesus when He was having astonishing success in prayer for healing. Notice His response after remarkable success, with growing crowds of thousands clamoring for the chance to hear Him and experience healing prayer:

> *But Jesus Himself would often slip away to the wilderness and pray.*
> (Luke 5:16)

JESUS PUT INTIMACY WITH GOD IN PERSONAL, PRIVATE PRAYER WAY AHEAD OF INTENTIONAL PRAYER FOR HEALING IN PUBLIC.

In fact, the ability to accomplish any kind of *power encounter* in Christ rested on Jesus's discernment of the action of His Father's Spirit. That shows up in the very next verse.

> *One day He was teaching, and there were some Pharisees and teachers of the Law sitting there who had come from every village of Galilee and Judea, and from Jerusalem; **and the power of the Lord was present for Him to perform healing.*** (Luke 5:17)

Read 5:17 carefully, focusing on the words in bold type.

"The power of the Lord was present for Him to perform healing" means that someone was there and noticed a tangible increase of power that was landing on Jesus of Nazareth. Those who witnessed this told Luke, who penned the third gospel; he confirmed the information and wrote it down for our learning.

The important inference lies in what the text doesn't say directly, but clearly implies.

THE POWER OF THE LORD TO PERFORM HEALING WASN'T ALWAYS PRESENT. JESUS WAS AWARE OF, AND COOPERATED WITH, "THE POWER OF THE LORD...TO PERFORM HEALING."

Why did Jesus pray? It does seem odd, since He was God the Son.

He prayed because He was also *the Son of Man*.

As the Son of Man, Jesus prayed to become aware of those moments when there was a healing anointing upon Him to even be able to get it done.

The author of the Gospel of Luke and the Acts of the Apostles makes a summary statement at the beginning of his gospel. Luke is the one gospel writer who tells us his methodology to write out the scrolls of Jesus's life. He was careful to make diligent inquiry. He gathered eyewitness testimony, investigated his facts, and did everything in his power to write down the events of Jesus's ministry in consecutive order:

> *Since many have undertaken to compile an account of the things accomplished among us, just as they were handed down to us by those who from the beginning were eyewitnesses and servants of the word, it seemed fitting to me as well, having investigated everything carefully from the beginning, to write it out for you in an orderly sequence, most excellent Theophilus; so that you may know the exact truth about the things you have been taught.* (Luke 1:1–4)

This means that Luke talked to the people who were there.

Someone saw this event in Luke 5—someone told Luke that there was a tangible increase of the *"power of the Lord"* resting on Jesus of Nazareth to bestow on Him the ability to heal the sick. The people in the room became aware that something was afoot, that healing power was present. *They felt the anointing.*

Luke heard the eyewitnesses talk about this, diligently compared their accounts, made notes, and wrote down this narrative in the order in which it happened. The conclusion is straightforward:

Jesus was "present" to the Presence!

It is blunt all through John's gospel. Here are two examples from Jesus's ministry, the first referring to a healing and the second to His role as the resurrected Judge:

Truly, truly, I say to you, the Son can do nothing of Himself, unless it is something He sees the Father doing; for whatever the Father does, these things the Son also does in the same way. (John 5:19)

I can do nothing on my own. As I hear, I judge, and my judgment is just, because I seek not my own will but the will of him who sent me.
(John 5:30 ESV)

Christ cooperated with those moments in which He sensed the *"healing power of God"* (Luke 5:17 MSG) landing upon Him. This was why He was aware when the woman with the hemorrhage touched His robe and the power flowed! (See Mark 5:30.)

Matthew, Mark, and Luke all reported the same phenomena: people sensing a flow of power, moving even through the Lord's clothing, and there was a longing among the weak, the sick, and the helpless to reach out and be put in contact with the healing stream.

> TO GET TO THAT PLACE OF HEALING PRAYER,
> IT WAS REQUIRED THAT JESUS PRAY! AND SO HE DID.
> JESUS PRAYED—ALONE IN SOLITARY PLACES
> AND WITH OTHERS.

Bear in mind that Jesus was from a prayer-saturated culture; in the rhythm of ordinary Hebrew life, every man, woman, and child took time to pray at least three times a day. When Luke 5:16 indicates that Jesus went off alone to pray in the wilderness, this was over and above the structured times of prayer built into an ordinary Jewish day. He needed to be alone with His Father for times of undistracted devotion.

We see the same practice at the beginning of His ministry in the Gospel of Mark. Note the enormity of the crowds, Jesus's healing prayer ministry, and His focused, consistent practice of time alone with God:

When evening came, after the sun had set, they began bringing to Him all who were ill and those who were demon-possessed. And the whole city had gathered at the door. And He healed many who were ill with various diseases, and cast out many demons; and He would not permit the demons to speak, because they knew who He was. And in the early morning, while it was still dark, Jesus got up, left the house, and went away to a secluded place, and prayed there for a time.

(Mark 1:32–35)

He started to pray for the entire town when the sun set, and then He got up early to pray by Himself!

If Jesus needed to pray to be *present to the Presence,* how much more do *we* need to pray? We need to do as Jesus did.

PERSONAL PRAYER TIME

Carve out a time in advance of the healing prayer time and reexamine your current habits in all areas of life.

If you are considering being part of a healing prayer team, the first step is to ensure that you have a regular devotional life by yourself and with others. Make a commitment to daily personal prayer. Lock it in your planning schedule, and then do it.

Make a commitment to meet regularly with a small group for biblical study, prayer, and accountability to help you grow spiritually.

Examine your walk with those you know and the God you love. Here are some starter questions to help you prepare and have a consistent walk with God. If you get through two of them now, as you read this, you will have done well!

+ Is your walk with God sweet or distracted? If the latter, ask for God focus.

+ Is there anyone who has anything against you? Plan to mend this if possible.

+ Is there anything between you and your Maker? If so, confess and repent.

+ Are your motives pure or is something else at work? Name this before the Lord.

+ Do you need to make things right with someone, confess a wrong, or make amends? Are you overstretched, overcommitted, burned out, or exhausted? Reexamine your planner and build in time for Sabbath.

+ Is there something God is putting in your heart? Name it, write it down, and ask God if there is an action step needed.

On the day before the prayer for healing appointment—and then a second time, just before interceding for another—prepare yourself for what lies ahead. You may practice this approach or develop your own form of preparation:

+ As you get ready to pray, relax your body through deep breathing or some other relaxation technique.

+ Open your Bible (or Bible app) to a favorite text and *be still before the Word*. Let God's peace rule in your heart. Let the Holy Spirit's Presence grow gently within you as you reflect on the Word. Let the Lord bring things to mind—an unexpected thought, a biblical text, or a picture of the person you are praying for. Whatever surfaces in your praying, make sure to pay attention to His interior Presence.

+ Allow the quiet of the Holy Spirit to focus your mind beyond any concerns except what God brings about in the prayer interchange.

+ Dwell in the healing Presence and power of Jesus, using Scripture to shape your praying. I (David) read 1 John 1:5 and 1:7 to picture the light of Christ and place myself and the person I am praying for in it.

God is Light, and in Him there is no darkness at all…If we walk in the Light as He Himself is in the Light, we have fellowship with one another, and the blood of Jesus His Son cleanses us from all sin..

(1 John 1:5, 7)

After repeating the Scripture, I picture Christ's light entering me as I breathe in and any darkness departing my body as I breathe out.

Maxie loves to use the phrase, "Christ in me—the hope of glory" (from Colossians 1:27) as he breathes to focus himself on God's Presence.

Here are some additional steps you can take to prepare for intercessory healing prayer:

- Call to mind Jesus's prayer for us *"that the love you* [Father] *have for me may be in them and that I myself may be in them"* (John 17:26 NIV).

- Deliberately place yourself in the company of the Holy Spirit, asking God to cleanse your conscious and subconscious mind of attitudes or thoughts that separate you from union with Christ, allowing God's grace and love to flow through you. Permit no reservation to limit believing faith. Deliberately invite the Holy Spirit to join you to the power, grace, and holiness of the risen Christ. Allow the Holy Spirit to birth faith for a new beginning within you.

Do this fully a day in advance of the designated time for public prayer. You may need to consider doing this for several days to attune your spirit with God's Spirit, so that the Spirit may pray through you.

You may wish to purchase a notebook so you can write down what comes to you as you pray. Some find that writing their praying helps them to focus on the Lord more easily. Use any method we have suggested until you discover how best to be prayerful using your own approaches.

PRAYER APPOINTMENT PREPARATION

In preparation for a public time of healing prayer, consider the setting and what steps should be followed under various eventualities:

1. As much as possible, make sure everyone feels at home. In a hospital setting, attempt to time the prayer right after a physician or nurse is scheduled to check on the person to minimize interruption. Ask those receiving prayer if they are more comfortable at home or in another setting, such as an altar at the front of a sanctuary.

2. In a service of healing prayer, the leader will indicate that what is shared in a prayer team's ministry will be kept confidential. (Make clear, however, that cases of abuse should be reported to the proper authorities.)

3. *Before* the start of the prayer appointment, ask if the person consents to having the prayer team place their hands on the person's shoulders, back, or head, and whether the person gives permission for anointing or dabbing with oil. Respect their wishes without pressure or question. Remember that there are people, particularly abuse victims, who are not comfortable with any touching at all. If the person says "no," simply pray without touch; the power and Presence of God are still present.

4. Make this commitment in advance: If a matter is sensitive, intercede only with their express permission. Ask if the team may pray into any sensitive matter. If they say "no," honor their wishes; do not further traumatize them by speaking what they are yet unable to hear said aloud. Sometimes healing unfolds over time.

5. If you are unsure how to proceed, communicate that it would be wise to speak with a pastor or an experienced intercessor.

THE PRAYER APPOINTMENT

When you are interceding for someone, be specific in your request to God. This means you must get clarity from the person for whom you are praying. Don't be in a hurry. Again, be totally present to the person for whom you are going to pray. Sometimes it is helpful to remind people of Jesus's question to blind Bartimaeus: *"What do you want Me to do for you?"* (Mark 10:51). Even if the need seems obvious to you, it is clear that Jesus made a blind man tell Him that he wanted his sight! Jesus asked the man to name his desire before He prayed for him. Sometimes there may be something you don't see or anticipate. Sometimes people need to be able to say out loud what it is they want God to do for them.

It is helpful to be aware of the possibility that a person who comes for prayer may be wrestling with God. If team members feel prompted, it is appropriate to ask questions such as, "Are you satisfied with your relationship with God?" or "Have you said 'yes' to following Jesus and asked the Holy Spirit to empower you to live like Jesus?"

If they indicate they are not connected with Christ, ask if they would like to be. Many will say yes. Lead them in a prayer of accepting Christ or being made new by the Holy Spirit. Then pray for the specific need for which they have come.

Invite the person to share what is going on in their life that prompted their need for prayer, then listen. Sometimes, as you listen and observe the person requesting prayer, a prompting may come to you that is not verbalized, such as a picture, a word, some Scripture passage, or a name. Be sensitive to this. It could be that God's Spirit is longing to pray through you. (See Romans 8:26–27.) Should you sense a strong prompting, simply mention it to the person without judgment; tell them what you are sensing and ask, "Does this mean anything to you?" If the one receiving prayer offers no response, gently lay aside what you felt, since it could have been your own longing or inclination for them. Yet if there is some kind of reply to what you have indicated, a different kind of response is needed from you.

Pay attention to emotions and feelings in youself and in the person for whom you are praying. In healing prayer, the person's body often responds with weeping, shaking, visible signs of peace and joy, or some kind of physical improvement, even as you pray, should God grant this. Pray into any kind of response that arises from your praying. Physical sensations sometimes accompany prayer for healing, in either the intercessors or in the one receiving the prayer. You are, after all, asking God to heal their body, mind, soul, and spirit.

EXPECT GOD'S INTERVENTION

Invite the person receiving the prayer to tell you what is in their heart or what is taking place in the affected area of their need. Jesus asked the blind man what was happening with his vision while He was praying and then prayed a second time. (See Mark 8:22–26.) If Jesus of Nazareth can ask what is happening in an afflicted area, discover that more intercession is needed, and then pray a second time, so can we!

Then petition the Lord to enable you and the one for whom you are praying to be open and receptive to God's Presence. Do not hurry the intercession. Wait upon the Lord as you pray. Then pray a clear, forthright petition, naming aloud whatever leading you have received based on the person's clear request. Speak out your God-honoring desires for the person's healing.

WHEN YOU HAVE CLARITY ABOUT THE PERSON AND THEIR NEEDS, BEGIN YOUR PRAYER BY ACKNOWLEDGING THE POWER AND GLORY OF GOD, FATHER, SON, AND HOLY SPIRIT.

There comes a moment when an increase of God's Presence occurs— usually a significant sense of compassion, rising peace, or a yearning to see something accomplished. Follow the leading you receive and pay attention to the Presence increasing or decreasing. Pray until the anointing lifts.

Should you receive no internal prompting, simply indicate that you are asking God for a blessing on them. Do not pretend or work up what isn't there. If you have no sense of any kind of intervention, simply tell those who are receiving your praying that God is at work. This does not depend on our interior senses always engaging. It depends on God.

Then ask the one receiving the healing prayer whether there is anything they would yet like to place before the Lord. Honor their "yes" by praying exactly as they have indicated. Honor their "no, we are done" by closing in a time of thanksgiving.

Close your prayer time by acknowledging that you and the person for whom you are praying are receiving the grace that God has offered. Express thanks for the grace received. Pray that you will go in faith certain of God's love, and that you are going to live in the strength of whatever healing power has been given. Proclaim to the Lord that you and those for whom you are praying will live in the reality of the abundance of Christ.

REFLECT AND RECORD

1. *"But Jesus Himself would often slip away to the wilderness and pray"* (Luke 5:16). If Jesus needed to slip away to pray and prepare Himself in prayer right after spectacular success in prayer for healing, what does this mean for you and me? What have you been learning lately in your practice of prayer?

   _____

   _____

   _____

2. Is there something that needs to be cleared away in your own heart before you pray for someone receiving intercession?

   _____

   _____

   _____

3. We should be specific in our praying:

   a. Pay attention to what the praying person is sensing, feeling, and thinking.

   b. Pay attention to what the one receiving prayer is sensing or feeling as well.

   What does this mean for the way you pray? Have you practiced being interactive while interceding for another person?

   _____

   _____

   _____

A PRAYER FOR READINESS

God, we give to You our limits and distractions but also our trust and availability. Do not let us withdraw at obstacles, but help us trust Your readiness to hear our prayers in any and all circumstances, whether ideal or unexpected. Teach us, as Jesus did, to regularly slip away even for a moment or two, to seek You on our own before seeking You for another. Teach us to respond to what You are doing for those we pray for and to move as Your Spirit moves on them and us together. Thank You for the grace of preparation. Amen.

12

PITFALLS TO AVOID, POTHOLES TO EVADE

Praying for others takes place in many different settings with many different people. Regardless of where you find yourself or who is asking for intercession, the following pitfalls are common ways that healing is misunderstood when it comes to prayer. Not only are they unhelpful in the work of intercession, but these misguided ideas can also inflict spiritual damage. Healing prayer is designed to bring people toward the love of God rather than distract them from it!

Wrong practices are like potholes on a highway. Progress can be inhibited or even stopped altogether when we develop practices that result in frustration rather than healing, adding a new layer of confusion, anger, isolation, or despondency.

Let's begin by remembering that we are *already/not yet* in our very lives, let alone in our times of healing prayer. We are *already* joined to Christ's fullness—but we are *not yet* completed and full in Him!

By now, it should be clear that the healing power of God is more than real! We are delighted when we see evidence that God intervenes directly… and we are perplexed when we see little or no evidence of any kind of effect arising out of the prayer. And yet we are still commanded to pray.

Sometimes we see healing. Sometimes we don't. We are simply not to know.

We commit to God, who sends anointings for healing prayer. This means that from time to time, when we do not sense the power of the Lord to perform healing, it is because we are not privy to the mind of God.

> *WE COMMIT TO LIVE FOR CHRIST. THIS MEANS WE LIVE IN "HOLY MYSTERY," AND GOD IS "WHOLLY MYSTERY."*

EIGHT WAYS HEALING PRAYER IS MISUNDERSTOOD

There are principles to safeguard our walk and then to make firm our commitment to praying as Scripture guides us. Watch out for these road hazards on the journey of learning to pray for healing.

1. DEMANDING THAT THE PERSON RECEIVING PRAYER HAVE MORE FAITH

Time and again, when obvious answers don't seem to come from praying, intercessors are tempted to believe the one seeking healing lacks faith. While God does use tenacious faith to accomplish both the mundane and the miraculous, Jesus didn't regularly speak this way. In fact, some are so worn down by despair that they have no resources left within them. The father of the demonized boy in Mark 9 had nothing left. He spoke with integrity when he said, *"I do believe; help my unbelief"* (verse 24).

Jesus didn't reprimand the father after he said that; He simply healed the boy based on His own faith, not the lack in the man.

No faith was exercised by the widow in the city of Nain when Jesus was moved to raise her deceased son. (See Luke 7:11–17.) We don't even know whether she believed or not, we only know she had lost her husband and her son. Jesus didn't ask her to believe more; He simply acted as the intercessor, following the leading He received.

On the other side of this, we find in John 11:1–44 that Mary and Martha did believe—and were horribly disappointed. They had spent good money sending servants to implore Jesus to drop everything and travel to them, based on His love for their brother. They asked Him to come quickly and heal their brother—and He didn't show up on time!

They believed and asked, based on their faith. Then Lazarus died, and their convictions were horribly wounded.

Jesus didn't tell them off. Rather, He acted in faith when they simply could not. They could not see what God was doing—and were brought to a place of joy when what God was planning occurred.

The intercessor, in this case the Lord, had faith when their faith had run out and they had none left!

2. REFUSING TO ACCEPT MEDICAL EXPERTISE ALONGSIDE OF HEALING PRAYER

As we point out throughout this book, medicine and miracle intertwine.

To say that they do not is a falsehood that would have been alien to the biblical authors. God has given us the creation to enjoy, to steward, and to explore. Those who investigate what is found in God's creation are acting as stewards of all God gave them. If someone dedicates fifteen years of their life to find a medicine to cure the disease that took the life of a family member or friend, accept the gift!

In Jesus's culture, oil was *medicine*. He anointed with oil and taught the apostles to do the same. (See Matthew 6:17; Mark 6:13; Luke 10:34.) Accepting medicine while seeking God's direct intervention is something that Jesus practiced. Both the benefits of modern medicine and the solace found in healing prayer are gifts of God; both are explored and practiced by people for the purposes of healing, health, and wholeness.

In chapter 4, we cited one example of medicine and miracle coming together—the healing of Hezekiah, king of Judah. (See Isaiah 38; 2 Kings 20:1–11.) Although we asked you then to examine this text and its implications, it bears repeating: King Hezekiah, one of the finest kings in Jewish history, received a prophetic word through Isaiah, one of the greatest prophets. The word was that the king would die, so he needed to get his house in order and attend to his final matters. Hezekiah prayed, telling God that he had led the Lord's people with a whole heart. God told Isaiah, *"Return and say to Hezekiah the leader of My people...'I will add fifteen years to your life'"* (2 Kings 20:5–6).

Then Hezekiah made a request that took nerve—he asked God to prove it!

Isaiah asked the Lord, and the king was granted a nature miracle: a shadow moving backward on a stairway. What is important for our purposes is to notice exactly what God did in this interaction around life, death, and healing prayer, involving one of the great prophets and one of the greatest kings in Jewish history. The healing was completed when the king received a medical treatment for his affliction: by the word of the Lord, Hezekiah was instructed to put a fig poultice over the afflicted area to suck out the poisons affecting his body.

He then celebrated the healing in a poetic writing. (See Isaiah 38:9–20.)

This account makes me (David) laugh, every time I read it! The king gets a major prophetic word, a second major prophetic word, and a nature miracle, and then he is told that he will get well when he *takes his medicine.*

Here, prophecy, prayer, a second prophecy, a promise of future heath, and medicine together in combination served as the agency of Hezekiah's healing.

THERE IS NO CONFLICT BETWEEN MEDICINE AND MIRACLE—AND GOD WILL GUIDE THROUGH WHATEVER IS GOING TO BE SENT OUR WAY!

3. BELIEVING THAT HEALING PRAYER IS AN INSTANT MECHANICAL PROCESS

Healing prayer is an interactive relationship between God, those being prayed for, and the intercessors.

In holy mystery, healing prayer can be simple or complex. Sometimes confession is needed. Sometimes a slight must be forgiven. Sometimes we are not to know the important factors, but must pray in faith, regardless of what we see or sense.

Sometimes healing occurs immediately as in the case of the leper of Mark 1:40.

Sometimes healing takes place when intercessors pray over a long season or in several times of repeated prayer, as Elijah did in praying for rain.

Sometimes partial healing is given and more prayer is needed. Jesus prayed twice to heal the blind man in Mark 8:22–26.

Sometimes there is demonic influence, as in the case of the bent-over woman in Luke 13:10–16.

Sometimes there are events that need to unfold in a life for the healing to be complete. Naaman the Syrian needed to submit to washing seven times in the Jordan River in 2 Kings 5:1–14 to be cured of his leprosy.

Sometimes God's answer is, "No. It is the appointed time for this one to come into my Presence," as when Jesus prayed in the garden of Gethsemane for another way, and God told Him "no."

The principle behind it all is summarized in two short sentences:

God initiates.

We respond.

Healing prayer is taught in James 5. After admonishing the congregation to the prayer of faith, with confession of sin, James cites Elijah the prophet as the paradigm for prayer for healing.

It is helpful to remember that Elijah spent three and half years of his life in a focused intercession. Then, at the decisive moment, Elijah prayed, and fire came down from the sky to burn up his offering to God. (See 1 Kings 18:38.)

And still there was no rain.

But within his spirit, Elijah heard *"the sound of abundance of rain"* (1 Kings 18:41 NKJV). He instructed the king, who had also been waiting for rain, to have a feast.

Elijah then went off and prayed in seven separate incidents, asking God for rain to fall on the land—and it did, after six attempts that yielded no results!

Remember, the prophet had already spent three years praying about that very drought, called down fire from the sky, and then was required to pray seven separate times to *pray in* the rain that God had already promised to send. This praying is the example used by James to illustrate how we are to accomplish prayer for healing. (See James 5:13–18.)

Even in the ministry of Christ, healing accounts vary. As we have already seen, on one occasion, Christ prayed twice because total healing did not come instantly. (See Mark 8:22–26.) In another, when Jesus met ten leprous men, in keeping with Mosaic law, He instructed them, *"Go and show yourselves to the priests"* (Luke 17:14)—to verify their healing before it had even taken place! They were healed while on their way.

Here is a personal example of a long interactive process coming to resolution over a period of years. While writing this book, I (Maxie) received this letter from my son, Kevin:

Pop,

Remembering the beginning of our pilgrimage.

We washed each other's feet and haven't looked back. Now the picture is so much more complete. Redemption, reconciliation, forgiveness, peace and a deep sense that "all is well."

Thank you for teaming up with me on this long journey. Thank you for giving me the security and confidence that I will survive and that I will thrive in this life if I hang on to the "garment of Christ"—faith!

I do and I am thankful you and I did and are on this pilgrimage together.

Kevin's reference to our washing each other's feet was significant. I had been called home from our major denominational meeting because

Kevin was in trouble. He had lived a roller-coaster life, involving drugs and alcohol, erratic and irresponsible living. When I arrived at his apartment, responding to the call, he came out with a basin of water and a towel, saying he wanted to wash my feet in gratitude for our love and prayers for him and his renewed commitment to Christ.

Needless to say, I also washed his feet.

That was at least twenty-five years ago. The journey has not been smooth, but his letter testifies to his healing and wholeness now. And so does his life.

Just recently, my wife Jerry and I were visiting with Kevin. He has a shelf in his kitchen on which he keeps his *precious things*. Among the pictures and other mementos, I saw a carving...and remembered. Around the same time that Carlos Velasquez had carved the praying hands that Jerry and I keep in the place where we pray each morning, Carlos promised to pray with us for Kevin and to carve something for him. I had forgotten, but there it was: a carving of the Good Shepherd, carrying a rescued lamb over his shoulders. Kevin passed through the kitchen as I was holding the carving. He smiled broadly and indicated that he was the rescued lamb.

I was reminded dramatically that we can't place a timeline on how and when our prayers are answered, but we must pray with the confidence they *will* be answered.

Prayer for healing does not follow a regimented approach with a strict formula for wrapping up in quick, tidy conclusion. As Pete Greig says:

> Prayer can be a lot like domino toppling, because while some prayers get answered the very first time you ask, most take months or even years of faithful asking before there is any kind of breakthrough. Day after day, you say essentially the same thing to God, and sometimes you wonder if it's ever going to make a difference. Then, one day, you pray the same thing you have prayed countless times before and, in a matter of minutes, it triggers the fulfillment of years of faithful prayer.[30]

---

30. Pete Greig, God on Mute: Engaging the Silence of Unanswered Prayer (Grand Rapids, MI: Baker Books, 2007), 181.

4. BELIEVING THAT SICKNESS IS ALWAYS A CONSEQUENCE OF SOMEONE'S SIN

In John's gospel, we read Jesus's view about the relationship between sin and someone's sickness or physical challenge:

As he went along, he saw a man blind from birth. His disciples asked him, "Rabbi, who sinned, this man or his parents, that he was born blind?" "Neither this man nor his parents sinned," said Jesus, "but this happened so that the works of God might be displayed in him."

(John 9:1–3 NIV)

The disciples assumed they knew why people were born with disabilities or infirmities; they believed that some ugly sin had to be the cause. They saw the blind man, and they wanted to know where that blindness came from. (And so do we!) In perplexity, they put forward the popular thinking of the day: they asked Jesus whose sin had caused this condition—the man's own sin or his parents' transgressions.

Jesus rejected their assumption altogether—and so should we.

In a fallen world, disease and illness exist. Many faithful believers have endured great physical illness along with hardship. Elisha the prophet died of an illness. (See 2 Kings 13:14.) Epaphroditus, who was sent to help Paul in prison, *"was sick to the point of death, but God had mercy on him"* (Philippians 2:27). Even Paul himself became extremely ill and fell sick among strangers—and that is how the church in Galatia was birthed. (See Galatians 4:13–14.)

There is no record of Elisha getting sick as a result of sin. Neither is there any word about Epaphroditus being anything other than a delightful servant of Christ, sent at great sacrifice and risk to help Paul while in prison. There is no evidence that Paul sinned in Galatia and then got sick as a result, only to receive care from strangers who became the core of a new church plant. In fact, he did signs and wonders there, according to Galatians 3:5.

While some illness can arise from risky behavior—for example, lung cancer from smoking and sexually transmitted disease from acting outside of God's provision for sexual expression in marriage—most illness is *not* a consequence of sin.

> *TO SUGGEST THAT SOMEONE'S ILLNESS, DISEASE, OR PHYSICAL CHALLENGE RESULTS FROM SIN IS BOTH SPIRITUALLY IMMATURE AND UNBIBLICAL.*

Even if a sickness arose from a sinful behavior, the gospel teaches us that Jesus saves us from sin. He desires our complete wholeness, regardless of our background. Remember, He didn't condemn either the woman at the well, who was living with her sixth partner (after five failed marriages), nor the woman caught in adultery. (See John 4:10 and John 8:11, respectively.) The implication is that Christ will heal regardless of our background. He isn't keeping score to determine our worthiness!

Prayer for healing requires kindness and gentle care.

In the vast majority of cases, people present themselves for healing prayer in a complex web of life. Many factors are involved in each prayer event, including genetics, age and stage, disease, an accident or injury, a quirk of anatomy, social or culturally acceptable behaviors, family background, medical error, addiction, and perhaps even the memory of an awful sin they now regret. This may be added to many other causes. Each prayer concerning a whole, complex person is unique.

This is why we need to be led by the Holy Spirit in our praying.

5. ATTRIBUTING ALL DISEASE TO DEMONIC ACTIVITY

Jesus did not usually talk this way. There are a *few* cases in the New Testament in which demonization and illness overlap, but they are not ordinary.

With a few exceptions, Jesus usually treated sickness as arising from a fallen world. He discerned whether someone was merely physically sick or whether there was a demonic influence and acted accordingly.

When dealing with a demonic influence, a pastoral leader should be invited to take part. In such instances, it is wise to set apart time for prayer and fasting. The use of a prayer team involved in intercession is the best course of action. Once again, the principle is clear: praying for the sick should be done in teams.[31]

6. ATTRIBUTING ILLNESS TO GOD

There is no New Testament indication that an illness or a disability is a *cross* for us to bear. Scriptures that refer to us picking up our cross refer to suffering rejection as disciples of Christ— and choosing obedience to Christ ahead of everything else in all circumstances. Jesus always healed disease; He never told people to accept that nothing was going to change, or that their diseases came from God. Disease is described as an enemy— and *"the last enemy that will be abolished is death"* (1 Corinthians 15:26).

7. GIVING UP EARLY, DECIDING CIRCUMSTANCES MUST JUST BE "DESTINY"

Surrendering to the grace and goodness of God is different from giving up in intercession out of frustration or discouragement. Quitting is not an option. Followers of Christ learn perseverance in prayer; we are compelled to choose life, seek healing, and trust that God is active in every situation in which we are earnestly and prayerfully involved.

8. TELLING THE AFFLICTED PERSON WHAT THEY CAN SAY OR NOT SAY

Much damage is done when we tell others that they are not allowed to say that they are quite ill or struggling emotionally, mentally, or spiritually. Frequently in Scripture, the affected person named their affliction to the intercessor. In one case, Jesus asked a blind man He had prayed for whether his eyesight was restored. When the man said he had received a partial healing, Jesus prayed a second time. He was not told to keep saying he was healed. (See Mark 8:22–26.) No one in the entire canon of Scripture used this approach.

---

31. Two resources are helpful with this: Francis MacNutt, *Deliverance from Evil Spirits: A Practical Manual* (Grand Rapids, MI: Chosen Books, 2009); and Peter J. Bellini, *The X-Manual: Exousia—A Comprehensive Handbook on Deliverance and Exorcism* (Eugene, OR: Wipf and Stock, 2022).

Rather, should a gift of faith be given—to trust God to work in what seems to be an impossible situation—the person with that gift will have complete assurance that God is at work in their *impossibility* and live accordingly in calm acceptance. This is very different than a demand that anyone who wants to be well must *stick to their confession* to activate God's healing power. No one in the Bible demanded a confession of a healing when it was not there. Jesus didn't do this, nor did Paul, Peter, Elijah, Elisha, Moses, nor anyone else.

> *IF NO ONE IN THE BIBLE DEMANDED A CONFESSION OF A HEALING, NEITHER SHOULD WE!*

God can be trusted to do something amazing with our praying. When we are praying, God carries the burdens of our deepest heart and brings them to the cross of Christ to send an answer, carried back by the Holy Spirit.

REFLECT AND RECORD

1. Healing prayer is interactive. We have previously noted that Jesus prayed twice to heal a blind man. Now let's take a look at the exchanges between the blind man, his friends, and Jesus:

   > *And they came to Bethsaida. And some people brought a man who was blind to Jesus and begged Him to touch him. Taking the man who was blind by the hand, He brought him out of the village; and after spitting in his eyes and laying His hands on him, He asked him, "Do you see anything?" And he looked up and said, "I see people, for I see them like trees, walking around." Then again He laid His hands on his eyes; and he looked intently and was restored, and began to see everything clearly. And He sent him to his home, saying, "Do not even enter the village."*
   > (Mark 8:22–26)

Did Jesus use a method to heal the man? What approaches did the Lord use in seeking God for this one's healing? How did Jesus pray for this man?

_____

_____

_____

What might this mean for your praying?

_____

_____

_____

2. Medicine and miracle intertwine. Do you have a story of a time when you sought both medicine and the healing power of God?

_____

_____

_____

A PRAYER FOR GUIDANCE IN HEALING PRAYER

Jesus, You did not belittle those who came to You for prayer. You saw each person and loved them as You prayed for their healing. Each healing prayer was crafted to suit the one in need. Show us how to let You guide our praying beyond our own assumptions. Train us to interact with those we pray for with simple joy and humility each time we pray. Amen.

13

GOD INITIATES, WE RESPOND: PRAYING INTO HOLY MYSTERY

Mystery surrounds all of our praying, particularly our intercession. Not long ago, I (Maxie) received a thank-you note from an old friend of mine who had suffered much. It contained a phrase that summarizes our intention in writing this resource:

"Embrace the mystery."

We all have questions! Why are some people healed when we pray, and others are not? Why are the prayers of some persons more effective than others? And perhaps the most perplexing and persistent question: Why are some prayers answered, and others are not?

We should not allow our questions to limit or shape our intercessions. Remember, Jesus Himself did not heal anyone independently of the Father's initiative. During His ministry, amazing miracles of healing had taken place. Yet when He returned to His hometown in Nazareth, His ministry was hindered because the people were offended by Him. Their familiarity bred contempt! Jesus Himself was astonished at the unbelief in His hometown and its effect:

And He could not do any miracle there except that He laid His hands on a few sick people and healed them. And He was amazed at their unbelief. (Mark 6:5–6)

We can make a strong case that the collective group unbelief of the crowd interfered with believing faith—an awful proposition! Yet even taking this singular account into consideration, we are still left with the one reality.

> *THE MYSTERY THAT SURROUNDS ALL OF OUR PRAYING, PARTICULARLY OUR INTERCESSION, IS PERVASIVE. IT WAS EVEN EVIDENT IN THE LIVES OF THE EARLY CHRISTIANS.*

Think of Paul, certainly one of the greatest healers in the early church. What mystery! His ministry of healing was so well-known that when handkerchiefs and aprons that had touched Paul were taken to the sick, *"the diseases left them and the evil spirits went out"* (Acts 19:12).

And yet when Paul needed his friends to share in ministry, he could not heal them.

+ Epaphroditus almost died. (See Philippians 2:25–27.)

+ Paul had to leave Trophimus sick in Miletus. (See 2 Timothy 4:20.)

+ Timothy, Paul's spiritual son, was frequently ill. (See 1 Timothy 5:23.)

+ Paul himself had a severe illness that kept him in Galatia, so he planted a church there. (See Galatians 4:13–14.)

Paul was left with *holy mystery* in these situations, as he was when he found no relief for his *"thorn in the flesh, a messenger of Satan to torment me"* (2 Corinthians 12:7). There is no consensus on what that thorn was; all we know is that Paul did not find relief after asking the Lord to remove it three times.

Even Christ walked in the reality of holy mystery because it surrounded *His* healing ministry too. In John 5, He heals a man who had been paralyzed for thirty-eight years. Obviously, some friends had brought him to the Bethesda pool, where he could be healed if he got into the water at the right time. He was among *"a multitude of those who were sick, blind, limping, or paralyzed"* (verse 3), but Jesus saw this particular man lying beside the pool and healed him instantly and completely.

The healing was grace to a despairing man—and we celebrate. Yet it leaves us with a question: Why did Jesus only heal *this* man when there were many others in exactly the same place? What about the others who were there?

There are accounts in the Gospels that say Jesus *"healed them all"* (Matthew 12:15; also see Matthew 8:16; Luke 6:19). Why did He not heal all of the other sick people at Bethesda?

Immediately after the healing of this one man, Jesus was involved in a theological dispute with religious leaders in which He gives us the principle that guided His whole ministry.

> *Very truly I tell you, the Son can do nothing by himself; he can do only what he sees his Father doing, because whatever the Father does the Son also does.* (John 5:19 NIV)

Jack Deere comments on this:

> Jesus healed only one person at the pool that day because his Father was only healing one person. If the Father was not healing, then Jesus could not heal. Jesus was completely obedient to the sovereign will of his heavenly Father for his entire ministry.[32]

Here we are brought face to face with the mystery: Jesus healed only one when countless other sick people were in that place seeking healing.

AFTER YEARS OF REFLECTION, WE EMBRACE THE REALITY THAT GOD INITIATES, AND WE RESPOND. IT IS GOD WHO DECIDES, AND GOD WHO HEALS.

The Gospel of Matthew gives us a summary of Jesus's healing ministry:

> *Jesus left there and went along the Sea of Galilee. Then he went up on a mountainside and sat down. Great crowds came to him, bringing the lame, the blind, the crippled, the mute and many others, and laid them*

---

32. Jack Deere, *Why I Am Still Surprised by the Power of the Spirit: Discovering How God Speaks and Heals Today* (Franklin, TN: Zondervan Reflective/Seedbed, 2020), 61.

at his feet; and he healed them. The people were amazed when they saw the mute speaking, the crippled made well, the lame walking and the blind seeing. And they praised the God of Israel.

(Matthew 15:29–31 NIV)

In Acts 3, God's power was demonstrated through Peter and John when a lame man was healed. News of this dramatic event spread, and a great crowd gathered in amazement. Peter was quick to remind the crowd that he and John had no power in themselves.

All the people were astonished and came running to them…When Peter saw this, he said to them: "Fellow Israelites, why does this surprise you? Why do you stare at us as if by our own power or godliness we had made this man walk? The God of Abraham, Isaac and Jacob, the God of our fathers, has glorified his servant Jesus."

(Acts 3:11–13 NIV)

It is God who decides and heals.

This gospel conviction, arising out of the plain teaching of the Bible, sets up the next account in this chapter as well as our closing chapter. Both accounts revolve around the theme of this book—that *healing prayer is God's idea*, and we are to *embrace the mystery*.

Pay attention as David shares some of the healing journey of his wife Elizabeth.

THE TESTIMONY OF ELIZABETH CHOTKA

We gave up, you know…

If memory serves, my wife and I prayed for this healing for around twenty years. We would see minor improvement, sometimes significant steps forward, only to see the affliction return. I can't tell you how many times this happened. Each time, hope would stir and then diminish, and we would grieve again. As one biblical writer, perhaps King Solomon, notes with great insight, *"Hope deferred makes the heart sick"* (Proverbs 13:12).

As time wore on, our hearts grew weary. It was easier not to pray, even though we were both still interceding for others with all manner of physical afflictions. We saw many restored to health, some instantly and against all odds. You have read some of their stories.

This did leave a strange taste in our mouths—yet God is God. And so, we determined to do something that now stands as a major principle in the way we understand prayer for healing:

Seek the Healer, not the healing.

Our prayers began before we were even married, when we were acquaintances and friends, fully two years before we decided to marry. Elizabeth was afflicted with a form of muscular dystrophy known as FSHD. Medical experts use one long word of this condition, but for ease of pronunciation, we have included hyphens: Facio-scapulo-humeral muscular dystrophy.

Elizabeth, her mom, her sister, and her niece all had this genetic disorder. For each of them, it meant that their faces and upper body limbs would become increasingly weakened. Their shoulder blades would move out of position, and chronic pain would be a daily challenge. Balance would become increasingly difficult, leading to dangerous falls. Back muscles would eventually wither away, making standing next to impossible. None of her family members with this syndrome were able to raise their arms above their shoulders.

Medical research indicates that FSHD is a "plateau, decline, plateau, decline" genetic disorder.

Damaged muscle tissue is not restored; instead, it becomes weaker. There is no known medical cure, only adaptive therapies leading to increasing dependency on mobility devices to assist with ordinary life.

When we started to sense attraction to each other, Elizabeth and I knew that our golden years would involve rapidly diminishing capacity, with the bulk of the physical work falling to me; most likely, that would include pushing a wheelchair. Yet she was the first woman to just accept me, let alone love me. She even laughed at my bad jokes! The love became reciprocal—and so we married.

But her decline accelerated with the birth of our son.

As is common with the onset of FSHD, Elizabeth was unable to raise her arms higher than her shoulders. By the time of our fifteenth wedding anniversary, if I was home, I had to lift her out of bed in the mornings so she could take a hot shower. The hot water made her limber and more mobile. I traveled on a regular basis, so when I was away, Elizabeth would have to set her alarm early so that she could function well enough to care for our two children. She would often trip and fall, damaging a muscle—and the decline would become more rapid.

It got to the stage where she had to walk with a cane, and moving from one place to another became harder for her. To get up the stairs in our home, she had to lift her leg with both hands, settle the leg on a step, take hold of the banister, pull herself up to the next step, settle her feet, and then repeat this for every step. It could take half an hour to get up to our bedroom.

We began to use a ramp for the entrance to our house and for the one step leading to the lower level. Elizabeth held onto a grocery cart to prevent falls while out shopping.

It was ironic that I would travel to teach people about prayer for healing.

Together, my wife and I had witnessed many astonishing, medically impossible healings. We would pray for others together and sense God's power flowing through us. Those people would become well, even while we were in emotional decline—and in Elizabeth's case, physical decline.

Then, my congregation partnered with two other churches to send teams to Uganda to help that nation rebuild after the devastations wrought by Idi Amin and Joseph Kony. Each year for three years, we brought work and teaching teams to Arua, Uganda, to help them rebuild their region and their nation. That town, the birthplace of Idi Amin, had been ravaged by both him and Kony. It had been a chronic war zone for twenty years.

The Ugandan bishop who organized several events there eventually came to speak in the congregation I was serving in Spruce Grove, Alberta, Canada.

Elizabeth and I had ceased praying about her health several years earlier; we were no longer seeking Jesus's healing. Rather, we were simply seeking Jesus and how best to serve Him with our diminishing strength.

During his visit to our church, the bishop preached about the Ugandan church's role in partnering with the government to remove Kony's brutally violent "Lord's Resistance Army." (Let's be clear: the Lord had *nothing* to do with that evil army, which was inspired by hell.) The bishop spoke of 300,000 intercessors praying in the streets of Kampala while the Ugandan army engaged Kony's army. Whenever the intercessors prayed, the Ugandan army prevailed. Whenever the Ugandan army didn't let the intercessors know they were fighting, Kony would put a curse on his attackers. They would freeze in terror and drop their weapons, which Kony then took.

The bishop shared stories of miraculous interventions and the power of God. It was an awe-inspiring series of messages. There was standing room only for our third weekend service. All of the seats were full, and people were lining the walls, so I sat on the steps leading up to the pulpit. Everyone was on the edge of their seats as the bishop shared one story after another of God's intervention in that conflict.

Suddenly, the man stopped preaching. He looked at me from my own pulpit, paused, and then looked down toward me again. Then, in his thick Ugandan accent, he said, "David! David! What is M.A.?"

I paused, caught off guard. I thought for a moment then said, "M.A.? Master of Arts? I don't know."

The bishop stopped and said, "No, something isn't right. I've got something wrong." Then he put his head on the lectern and prayed silently.

After a long pause—and of course, it seemed longer than it likely was—he looked up and said, "It is a wasting muscle disease. It starts in the head and neck. Your face sags, and it goes down into your shoulders and back. You lose your balance and get dizzy. You get tired easily. If you lose a muscle, it is lost forever, and you wind up in a wheelchair..."

The bishop continued describing the symptoms—nailing the exact medical trajectory for FSH muscular dystrophy—in front of 650 people in a packed sanctuary. Goosebumps traveled up and down my spine. He was describing my wife's symptoms as if he were reading them from a medical textbook. I am sure my eyes opened very wide, as the realization dawned on me.

I was looking at my wife, sitting right beside me, and watched something astonishing occur even as the bishop continued to describe her symptoms. That was when I heard him say:

"Whoever has these symptoms—Jesus has just healed you!"

Then, for the first time in over thirty years, sitting next to me, my wife raised her hands above her head—without pain or restriction. Later, she didn't even remember doing this because it happened automatically while she was focused on worshiping the Lord!

Then the bishop went back to preaching his message about Kony's defeat, as if it were a great inconvenience to him that God had interrupted his sermon!

We were astonished.

Close friends were sitting all around us, and they knew that what had happened was impossible. The congregation was also astonished.

And so was our doctor, who watched this closely for months and eventually wrote a note indicating that all outward marks of FSH muscular dystrophy had vanished. They have never returned—and that was fourteen years ago.

We truly knew that Elizabeth was fully healed when, without thinking, she ran up the stairs in our home about two weeks later.

The date of that transformative healing moment was February 22, 2009. It happened at 11:42 a.m. at Spruce Grove Alliance Church in front of 650 witnesses. Elizabeth has no sign of FSH muscular dystrophy in her body at all. A simple test verified the reality. Anyone with FSH cannot whistle because the facial muscles are among the first to deteriorate, and they cannot be shaped for that. However, my wife can whistle! In fact, from that day forward, she has regrown muscle tissue after any injury—a medical impossibility with FSHD.

We sought the Healer, not the healing.

And after two decades of seeking Him, the healing came when we had abandoned all hope that the gift would be granted.

Embrace the mystery.

We have learned that we can't demand miracles; we can only cooperate with the Lord when He sends them our way. There are mysteries and unanswered prayers for many we know and love. Why is one healed and another not? Why did this one take more than twenty years? These questions fall into the category of *holy mystery*, a mystery that calls us to seek the Healer all the more profoundly.

Elizabeth and I are forever grateful to the Lord for this astonishing, medically impossible blessing. This was genetic transformation, the most incredible healing event we have ever witnessed.

Jesus is the Healer. And His healing gifts continue, even into the twenty-first century. Should Jesus move upon you with the Holy Spirit and fill your heart with fire as you think about praying for another—well, pray!

WE CAN'T DEMAND A MIRACLE, BUT WE CAN PARTNER WITH GOD AND COOPERATE WHEN HE DETERMINES TO SEND ONE.

We were granted to know the other side of the verse from Proverbs 13 that we cited earlier:

*Hope deferred makes the heart sick, but **desire fulfilled is a tree of life**.*   (Proverbs 13:12)

REFLECT AND RECORD

1. Jesus said these words after accomplishing a healing of the man by the pool of Bethesda:

    *Very truly I tell you, **the Son can do nothing by himself**; he can do only what he sees his Father doing, because whatever the Father does the Son also does.*   (John 5:19 NIV)

    Jack Deere indicated that this text made this truth plain:

    Jesus healed only one person at the pool that day because his Father was only healing one person. If the Father was not healing, then Jesus could not heal. Jesus was completely obedient to the sovereign will of his heavenly Father for his entire ministry.[33]

---

33. Ibid.

Does this thought help you in attempting to understand healing prayer?

_____

_____

2. Paul's life was overflowing with significant signs of God's activity. Yet we know from Paul's own words that he could do nothing out of his own resources. He was only able to heal when God's Spirit granted him those gifts. Recall that his "fellow soldier" Epaphroditus almost died; Paul had to leave sick Trophimus in Miletus; his spiritual son, Timothy, was frequently ill; and Paul himself planted the church in Galatia because he was severely ill there. What does this mean for how we understand healing prayer?

_____

_____

3. Both Maxie and David have learned a singular principle in prayer: *God initiates, and we respond.* When the anointing of the Lord is upon us, God's power through us can accomplish anything. When the anointing is not guiding, we are unable to do anything. This leads us to a call to *embrace the mystery.* Does this approach help in the way you pray?

_____

_____

A PRAYER TO BE LED

Father, we know what it is to be led. And we know when we have simply fallen on our own resources. The difference is profound. Jesus did nothing unless You showed Him. If Jesus could do nothing apart for Your guiding, we can do considerably less! So guide us! Lead us! Teach us to walk in Your power and to embrace the mystery. Amen.

14

LIVING BETWEEN THE TIMES— GROANING, GRIEVING, AND A GIFT OF JOY

If we were to attempt to put the New Testament into a single phrase, it would be that we are *"already/not yet…"*

That is exactly how it feels. We live between what we have *already* received in the gospel—salvation in Christ, and from time to time, wonders that flow from God's mercy—and what is *not yet* realized in full: an end to sorrow, sin, and death, our new bodies, the resurrection of the dead, a new heaven, and a new earth.

It is summarized in 1 John 3. The second verse is key:

See what kind of love the Father has given to us, that we should be called children of God; and so we are. The reason why the world does not know us is that it did not know him. Beloved, we are God's children ***now***, *and what we will be has* **not yet** *appeared; but we know that when he appears we shall be like him, because we shall see him as he is. And everyone who thus hopes in him purifies himself as he is pure.*

(1 John 3:1–3 ESV)

Did you see it in the text?

Now *that* is a grand finale that will fill us all with joy, energy, life, and delight. We suspect that anyone who loves Christ is filled with a yearning for that time.

> WE ARE GOD'S CHILDREN "NOW," BUT WE ARE "NOT YET" AS WE SHOULD BE. AT THE END OF TIME, WE WILL SEE HIM AND BECOME JUST LIKE HIM!

Yet we do live between those times. Sometimes we taste grace and see miracles, and other times our hearts are crushed with despair. There are bittersweet times when the future hope of the resurrection and the present reality of living in a place with trial and despair collide.

A BITTERSWEET TESTIMONY

Let me (David) tell you of one such time. I had a wonderful friend named Bob. I met him and his wife Marlene on my first pastoral call for the new church where I had just agreed to serve.

Bob was filled with cancer, and everyone was told he would soon die. I had just arrived in town, and someone in the office told me the couple had asked, "Oh, could our new pastor come and spend some time with us?"

So I got in the car and drove for twenty minutes to Bob's home in the countryside. When I was welcomed inside, I saw a man with oxygen tubes attached to his nose while his doting, loving wife did her best to care for the man she had pledged to love "till death do us part."

He had difficulty moving and breathing, so I pulled up a chair to sit close beside him. He had made his peace with God and wanted to sense consolation deep within. So I prayed for him, not knowing that the church elders were already about to travel to his home and pray as well. (I was very new, and we had not yet had our first elder meeting.) My time of prayer was gentle and understated. I read some Scripture and asked God to increase Bob's sense of Presence in that home.

Then I went home and told my wife that I would probably have to officiate at a funeral very soon.

When the elders gathered to pray a day later, something happened.

Everyone *felt* something. They *knew* that something had happened.

Two weeks later, Bob was golfing at Myrtle Beach, enjoying warm sunshine and laughter with a longtime friend. His cancer went into remission, and he began to regain the weight he had lost due to the ravages of the disease.

So began the healing prayer journey—a bumpy road for all of us, especially for Bob, his wife Marlene, and their two adult children.

We prayed a lot. Sometimes we were praying about important matters that had nothing to do with his health. Bob had become one of the elders in that church and was tasked with implementing a new evangelism program.

From time to time, we did pray about Bob getting completely well.

When cancer goes into remission, the medical community waits for years before saying the affliction has been defeated. So Bob was waiting for that word.

During another prayer time, Bob was filled to overflowing with the joy of the Lord. While my wife and I were praying with Bob and Marlene for him to become completely well, he bubbled over with laughter. He laughed for hours! He simply couldn't stop, nor did he want to stop.

After that, we all became friends. Not only did we learn together, taking part in a Billy Graham school of evangelism, but we also served together, and we chuckled together. He and Marlene joined my wife and I, together with two other couples, and we would get together about once a month to just laugh!

And laugh we did. Bob and Bill would exchange jokes, teasing, and gentle humor until all of us were hooting and sometimes letting out a deep guffaw or two. All four women were friends whether we were together as couples or not—and we would simply do a lot of *harmless nothings* together to let off steam.

Some of my fondest memories in life come from those times.

Then the tide turned. After about four years, Bob's cancer returned.

And of course, we responded as anyone would—we prayed, we fasted, we sought medical intervention, and we visited other churches whenever there was any kind of healing service. I distinctly remember driving an hour one way to get to the service in the church up the road. I noticed Bob's complexion had taken on an orangish hue. When I asked about this, he told us that he was drinking copious amounts of carrot juice—two or three full quarts a day!

And so, we laughed even about that…until the cancer started giving him unbearable pain. That affliction returned with a vengeance. Soon he was in hospital—and I was in the room when he drew his final breath, just a few seconds before his daughter arrived to sit with her dad.

We wept together—the family, the elders, the church, and our friends. You see, Bob was only fifty-five when the cancer took him. And all of us grieved that he had *passed before his time.*

I gave the funeral service, pronounced the familiar words as the casket was lowered into the ground, and gave the benediction. Then I went back to my office, closed the door, and sobbed uncontrollably, unable to understand why. Why had this godly, kind man, our *Bible-guy elder,* experienced a remission right after the elders had prayed, had it last for years, and then died young in excruciating pain! Why?

I had officiated at many funerals before this one. Some were for the very young, but most were for the very old. This one hit hard. I wasn't myself for quite a while.

Some weeks later, I was visiting with our friends, and all of them were thanking God—*for Bob's healing!*

I was stymied by that thought. Remember, I had just buried our friend!

When I asked what they meant, they all looked at me as if I should have known. Then they remembered that I had not known Bob as long as they had. Before Elizabeth and I came to town, the guys had been a threesome and had known each other for a full decade. So they filled me in on what I had missed.

Bob had been clinically depressed for more than ten years, and it had been far worse than a blue funk. He was unable to organize his life, let alone be a husband to his wife and a father to their two children.

He was spiraling down into deep despair when the cancer started. The depression predated the cancer by a dozen years. Bob had no energy and had not laughed, had fun, or experienced joy for years—until the elders prayed, just a day or so after I had arrived in town. Then, when we prayed together and he started to laugh, my wife and I were the only ones who did not know that he hadn't laughed like that in years and years.

Bob was healed of all vestiges of clinical depression all through his last five years—all the time I had known him.

Everyone who knew him before the elders prayed immediately knew that there had been a significant change. It was deepened in the prayer time with my wife and I when Bob started to laugh, but neither of us had a lonely clue that he had experienced an astonishing infilling of God-focused joy that would remain his defining personality trait for the remainder of his life.

Joy became the dominant center of his life, from that time of prayer with the elders until the Lord called him home. Bob's healing was *already* and *not yet*.

He was *already* healed of clinical depression. He was in remission for three years filled with laughter and love, as well as service in and for the Lord, until it became clear that he was *not yet* done with the cancer. Even so, he was well ready to meet his Savior when his time came.

We grieved and lamented the loss of our friend. Yet Bob loved the Lord, tasted grace, was granted years of healthy delight with his wife and two adult children, made his peace with God, and entered the Presence of the Lord by passing through death to life.

Paul, the apostle who suffered much, indicated that he had despaired even of life itself. (See 2 Corinthians 1:8.) Yet he prevailed to plant churches, preach the gospel, and write one-third of the New Testament before he was executed in Rome. He sums up *holy mystery* beautifully:

> *For we know that if the tent that is our earthly home is destroyed, we have a building from God, a house not made with hands, eternal in the heavens. For in this tent we groan, longing to put on our heavenly dwelling, if indeed by putting it on we may not be found naked. For while we are still in this tent, we groan, being burdened—not that we*

*would be unclothed, but that we would be further clothed, so that what
is mortal may be swallowed up by life. He who has prepared us for this
very thing is God, who has given us the Spirit as a guarantee.*

(2 Corinthians 5:1–5 ESV)

Once again, we are confronted with holy mystery. Medicine and miracle intertwine.

You may know this already. You may have tasted miracle and despair. Perhaps, just like Paul, you have looked to Christ for consolation when understanding ran out.

We look forward to the day when we will see Him and become like Him.

This brings us to an account of an *already/not yet* experience in the life of Maxie and a couple he was mentoring for ministry.

AN ALREADY/NOT YET STORY

I (Maxie) find great joy and meaning mentoring young clergy. Although most of the time it is informal, I have deliberately dedicated specific, formal time to what I see as a *calling*. I recently spent a year with eight young leaders who participated in a program of World Methodist Evangelism, mentoring them for one to two hours once a month via phone calls or Zoom.

The focus was Christian leadership. The secret of spiritual leadership is to attend to our woundedness and be a healing presence for the woundedness of others.

The dynamic that facilitates this best for the preacher is called *confessional preaching*. In our preaching, we must willingly open our lives to others and be transparent as a visible reminder of what the gospel is all about. This means that we must honestly be ourselves and share ourselves in all the uniqueness with which God has gifted us. This renders powerless the two enemies of vital spirituality: pretension and imitation.

I've had many memorable experiences during my more than seventy years of ministry, but the year with those eight young ministers was a treasure. Very early on, each one began to share deeply and revealingly. Prayer was an essential practice; they prayed for me, and I prayed for them and their work in differing congregations.

As I began to work with David on this book on healing prayer, the experience of Sarah, the only woman in our group, came vividly to mind. She and her husband are both ordained. He was not in the program, yet I feel like I know him and their son through what Sarah has shared. The mentoring program has ended, but I still keep up with them. I asked Sarah if I could share their experience in this book. She agreed, and it soon became obvious to me that it would be more personal and powerful if we shared it in her own words and way. Here is her deeply meaningful testimony—an *already/not yet* account of holy mystery:

SARAH'S TESTIMONY

When you pray, you don't imagine the long, winding road that may unfold in answered prayer. Whether we intend to or not, when we surrender to God in prayer, knees buckled beneath us in desperation, broken in spirit, and longing for God to move, we imagine asking something of God with urgency—and expect a timely reply.

The first of those prayers whispered in broken desperation came a lifetime ago. My husband and I were newly married, happily finding our way in life and ministry together. We'd gotten our feet under us as husband and wife and decided we were ready to have a family. We were in our late twenties, had secure jobs, had been married for a few years, and were certain we could handle a new chapter of growing in love together by loving and raising children. I'll never forget sitting alone in a doctor's office as the doctor flung open the door to my exam room and said without prelude, "You're infertile. It will be very difficult for you to get pregnant." I left, hiding my sobbing behind sunglasses and in total denial.

For more than a year, I lived as if that appointment didn't happen. Eventually, I found the courage to walk down a road I didn't want to walk and began working with a new doctor to have the family we longed for. A new doctor in a new community had more hope and believed I could get pregnant with help from a little pill. He was right. And fairly quickly, Gabe and I learned we were expecting our first baby...until we weren't. Before I could see them on a screen or hear their heartbeats, they were gone. And we began to experience a darkness that often suffocated us. I began to ask God with new desperation to give us what we longed for. We would regroup again, try again, and eventually get pregnant again, this time finding ourselves in the emergency room, desperately searching an ultrasound screen for the flicker of a heartbeat and hoping that this newly forming life would hold on despite what my body was trying to do. We did our best to put one foot in front of the other, trusting our doctors that miscarriage was "normal," and that I'd undoubtedly be pregnant again one day, successfully.

We began to share our suffocating grief with the congregations we led, asking for their grace, care, and strength in prayer to help us keep going and to intercede on our behalf. In our overwhelming darkness, I remember asking God for "just one baby." I told Him I didn't need a whole family like everyone else. Just one baby would do. I often pleaded in the way a child believes they desperately can't live without something. I would pull myself together between prayers of desperation to push through another sermon and another appointment.

In the months ahead, wondering how we were supposed to keep going after losing two precious babies, I would pray for direction and clarity, that God would help me know what to do. But I remember mostly praying for joy. The grief of eight years of painful infertility, the loss of two babies, and the all-encompassing, suffocating uncertainty and sadness caused me to pray for joy, begging for the transformation of my darkness to His incredible light. We would go on to lose a third baby later that year. And as our doctor grieved with us, in what seemed to be an answer to prayer in getting pregnant, but an unanswered prayer in pregnancy growing to the fullness of life, he pointed us to further treatment, one that would unearth the fullness of my infertility, but after months of treatment leave me empty-handed in ever getting pregnant again.

In the eight years of infertility and the pain of losing three babies, I white-knuckled to the promise of God's presence, declaring the truth that He was so near, even when I couldn't feel it. I often felt the ongoing uncertainty, wondering if or when God would give us the tangible thing we so desperately pursued. As I longed, hoped, and prayed, I reached the end of my rope. I couldn't take one more IV, one more doctor's appointment, or one more scan. I felt like I had been banging my head on a brick wall and finally admitted I'd never knock it down.

Several times during this painful journey, my husband, with compassion for my suffering and struggle, would offer the possibility of adoption to relieve our pain. I knew he wanted to help, but I couldn't hear it. I needed to exhaust all my efforts and do everything in my power so I wouldn't look back with regret if I came up empty-handed. But just as God had always been leaning into our darkness, He was ready when I finally laid that down. As I sobbed into my hands in my car, falling apart in my local Walmart parking lot—listening to a beautiful song of God's blessing in pain, wrestling through my struggle of wanting to carry a baby, and struggling to close that door for adoption—I heard the Lord say, "But I adopted you."

And with an overwhelming sense of humbling regret for my blindness and, simultaneously, God's incredible gentleness, my heart was changed, and God began to work in me. With this simple nudge, He began to heal me from those years of pain as we stepped into the uncertain journey of adoption. As we began to trust God to answer our prayer in unexpected ways, and as we surrendered our own way, God began to fling wide the doors and, less than a year later, place a beautiful baby boy in our arms that would be the delight and joy of our lives. We began to see that God had been working to answer our prayers with great mystery but with incredible accuracy to the many prayers we prayed. Our son would have the most contagious and joyful laugh ever heard. The first time I heard it, I knew God heard those many desperate prayers.

Once we held him in our arms, I never breathed another prayer for more. He was everything. Our family and our hearts were whole. God healed my heart with the incredible, mysterious gift of adoption, even though my body was never healed, and the mystery of death in me was never solved.

We watched him grow, soaked in every moment of this incredible life we had been given by such sacrifice, pressed forward in ministry, pursued education, and ran after all the beautiful things God had for us. Several years after we first held him, Gabe and I attended a special conference. One evening, I stood in worship, listening for what the Lord might say to me. At some point, I had a very rational thought and a strange sense of unease that in all my prayers for a baby, a family, and joy again, so many years before, I had never actually prayed that God would make me pregnant. It felt, at the time, like I had subconsciously avoided praying for pregnancy because I had been so devastated by miscarriage and infertility so early. If I had never prayed to be successfully pregnant, I couldn't have been disappointed if God didn't answer my prayer. I hadn't prayed for my healing, so I couldn't be hurt when I wasn't.

That night, so many years later, as I juggled those swirling thoughts, I decided to go forward for healing prayer as an act of trust, to ask God to give me something I wouldn't receive. They laid hands on my belly and asked God to fill it.

I returned to my seat in worship, my heart full from prayerful surrender. I lost myself as we sang in worship to the Lord. And then, the most unexpected thing happened. I had a vision. With eyes wide open, I saw Jesus standing in front of me, just a touch away. He was holding a baby. He looked down at the baby, looked up at me, and said, "She looks just like you."

I enjoyed the gift of His presence for just a moment, and then He was gone. I was surprised but deeply peaceful. And with the most casual curiosity, I turned to my husband, whispered in his ear, and said, "I just saw Jesus. Remind me to tell you about it later." I would fill him in on the vision in the hours ahead, and we casually wondered what it all meant.

In the days ahead, I wondered if it meant that God would give us a baby or if He was showing me that He held the precious babies we lost, giving us a glimpse of our coming reunion. I held onto the vision the way Mary "treasured these things in her heart" as a precious gift.

Once again, I returned focus to life and ministry and told our story as often as possible so those walking in the darkness of infertility, miscarriage, and grief might find hope in knowing they aren't alone and find strength in hearing how God can be present in their pain.

I lost track of the years between, how much time passed between prayers and visions, of seeing Jesus but not seeing anything miraculous after such an incredible vision that was now a faded memory.

One day, more than two years later, I grew frustrated with some pain I had been experiencing. I had been uncomfortable for a while and hadn't found relief in waiting it out or typical medications. So one Monday morning, I decided to call a doctor to find relief. After a decade of infertility, and now well beyond forty, I didn't think I was pregnant. But I grabbed a pregnancy test as an act of declaration that my God certainly had the power to heal if He desired, having just preached a sermon on the miraculous pregnancy of Elizabeth the day before. And with a numbing sort of surprise, I quickly saw the infamous double lines and nudged my husband as he walked groggy-eyed into the bathroom, saying, "You might want to look at that." With a surreal numbness, I called the doctor's office that had helped us navigate so many miscarriages *twelve years* before. I told the receptionist my life story and my disbelief at what I saw that day.

In a sort of out-of-body experience, I went to my appointment. To my amazement, as soon as the tech switched on the ultrasound screen, I saw the familiar shape of a growing baby, heard the "whoosh" of a heartbeat, and learned that I was already ten weeks' pregnant.

Amazingly, completely, miraculously. That day, I knew we had received a divine gift.

Twelve years after our last loss. Ten years after receiving the incredible answer to prayer in the adoption of our son. Two years after seeing Jesus holding a baby and not expecting one, we were delighting in the gift of a miracle. That gift grew even sweeter as we told our son that he would be a big brother, that his secret prayers for a sibling had been answered, and we rejoiced in the baby girl that would make us an unexpected family of four.

As we delighted in the goodness of this gift, life kept moving on in the most unexpected ways.

It wasn't long before we found ourselves navigating uncertainty and trusting God with the gift He had given us as we learned our daughter would be born with Down's syndrome. Her diagnosis would shift our doctor's attention, and we would be placed under significant monitoring to watch her grow. Every day was a delight as she turned somersaults inside me and reminded me of the gift of life. In spite of two complex diagnoses—Down's syndrome and a congenital heart defect—we enjoyed a beautiful, joyful, easy pregnancy and anticipated her arrival.

Then, one hot summer day, I noticed our sweet girl was quiet. We debated what it might be and brushed off her stillness as anxiety from our previous pain. That night, I told myself to rest and wake up without worry.

But morning didn't bring the relief I hoped for. I had a profound sense that something else was wrong. I went to my room to lie down and gather myself. But as I closed my eyes, I found myself in prayer again. This time, in total desperation, asking God to heal her, to wake her up, and give her fullness of life. Though I couldn't verbalize it in prayer, I had a sense she was gone, and I was asking the Lord to show up with the same miraculous power by which He had given her to me, with the same power He had revealed Himself in this pregnancy, and to give life to the gift *He* had chosen to give me.

In a way I can't possibly explain, the Lord was profoundly silent but powerfully present. I could feel Him, almost see Him. As I lay there, weeping and praying, I sensed His eyes downcast, like He couldn't look at me. And I knew exactly what He was saying. His silence was everything as if, in His great compassion, He couldn't bring Himself to tell me she was gone. Three weeks before she was supposed to come home, we lost her. I lay quietly weeping in my bed while my son nervously tried to entertain himself in the living room among piles of boxes from our move just hours before. I gathered myself, told Gabe what was wrong, and planned to leave for the emergency room.

In our unfolding darkness, the Lord was present arranging our care. I was swept right back into labor and delivery emergency care. They searched for her heartbeat forever, watching her chest for any sign of life. But as soon as he laid the ultrasound wand on my stomach and her body appeared on the screen, I knew she was truly gone. Her little body was no longer twisting upside down in somersaults or playfully sleeping with her feet over her head; she was lifeless. They left me alone for a moment as I called Gabe and told him the news, as we talked through our options for delivering her, who could care for our son while we awaited her stillbirth, and how we would tell him. I called my mother, who cried and said, "We were so close." And the nurses wheeled me into a private room where we would begin bringing her body into the world. For two days, the doctors cared for me, helped my body with the process of stillbirth, and on June 16th, we held her beautiful, perfect body in our arms without reason or explanation for her death. We had the gift of seeing our beautiful daughter, holding her close, rocking her for a few hours as we grieved, admiring her features and weeping at the gift that seemed to slip through our grasp.

I write this nearly a year and a half after holding her in my arms. I've never attempted to put words to the story of her death, in part because they are a precious treasure, one that may be misunderstood. But I've struggled to document the story of her beautiful life and death because we're still walking through the mystery of unfulfilled healing. We hold in tension the miracle of *my* physical healing against the healing she *didn't* receive, the gift of life we received in my pregnancy against her death, and the lifeless body we held. We struggle to understand why God would give her to us but allow her to die. And we're learning to lean into the reality that God knows what may never be understood to us in this life.

We still don't know how her short life will be redeemed, but we trust it will. We know more than ever that God has heard every cry and been close in every darkness. We know the sweetness of His presence more profoundly because of the pain. We know Him more deeply because He revealed Himself in moments of great glory and in the dust and ashes too.

And in a way that's hard to understand, we're so thankful to have walked with Him in such a beautiful mystery.

The testimonies of both Sarah and Bob are clear cases of believers in the Lord tasting God's goodness and waiting for the day when we find *"Death swallowed by triumphant Life!"* (1 Corinthians 15:54 MSG).

REFLECT AND RECORD

1. Every life given over to God contains the elements found in this Scripture:

    *Beloved, we are God's children **now**, and what we will be has **not yet** appeared; but we know that when he appears we shall be like him, because we shall see him as he is.*   (1 John 3:2 ESV)

    Take a moment and write down the main point of this text, in two themes:

    a. *"We are God's children **now**,"* and that means:

    _____

    _____

    _____

    b. *"What we will be has **not yet** appeared,"* and that means:

    _____

    _____

    _____

2. Paul's words about groaning in our earthly tent, the human body, makes it clear that he experienced joy and trial too. (See 2 Corinthians 5:1–5.) Yet he insists that God prepares us by sending His Spirit. What does this mean for you?

_____

_____

_____

3. Sarah's story contains many ups and downs—miracle and despair as well as hope lost and hope reborn. What speaks to you from her testimony?

_____

_____

_____

A PRAYER TO BE THANKFUL

Lord, sometimes we see miracle and despair side by side. Yet we learn that mercy comes wrapped inside frail human bodies. Teach us to recognize that healing comes in many forms—and that a wounded spirit made whole is just as much a gift as a body made well. Teach us to be thankful in our earthly tent as we live between the times, living between our present life and our future hope. In Jesus's name! Amen.

15

ANY MIRACLE JESUS WANTS TO GIVE

There can be no question.

As we read the Gospels, we soon conclude that Jesus's ministry was (and is) a healing one. The New Testament healing stories are like dramatic exclamation points to the totality of Jesus's ministry. In this book, we have referenced many of those stories, including those that encompass emotional, mental, physical, and spiritual healing.

One of those stories is about a man in the region of Gerasenes. The demons within him called themselves *"Legion, for we are many"* (Mark 5:9). He was possessed of demons to the point that he was compelled to dwell among the tombs. He knew there were powers within him that really were not himself. He would often cut himself with stones because the demonic darkness in him brought on nightmares from which he thought he could never escape. These unclean forces within him were so powerful that he tore apart shackles and chains meant to bind him in order that he might not hurt himself or anyone else. No one could restrain him.

He screamed among the tombs as he eked out some shadow form of life among the gravestones of the dead.

And then it happened. Jesus came.

An unusual truth is found here. No matter how many demons there are or how strong they are, they cannot prevent someone who is afflicted or possessed from running *toward* Christ the Lord. This demonized man ran up to Jesus and bowed down before Him just as He was getting out of a boat. (See Mark 5:2, 6–7.) He ran toward the Lord even though he was infilled by unclean powers he could not control.

Jesus took authority over the dark powers controlling that man, cast them out, and spoke the healing word. The result is expressed in one of the most understated sentences in the New Testament:

> *And they came to Jesus and saw the demon-possessed man, the one who had had the legion, sitting there, clothed and in his right mind.*
>
> (Mark 5:15 ESV)

It is understatement to say that Jesus's ministry is a healing one.

The lovely parade of those healed by His miraculous power could go on and on. They were deaf, blind, dumb, and lame—but now, in the parade, they hear, they see, they shout praise to God with their loosened tongues, and they leap with joy because they've been healed.

You can't read any one of the Gospels without coming to the conclusion that Jesus's ministry not only contains healing, but *is* a healing one. For the most part, in this book, we have focused on more than physical healing, and much of that has been *miraculous*. We are insistent in our conviction that the miraculous is not divorced from the medical. Previous chapters have included two of David's stories in which miracle and medicine were dramatically intertwined.

IT IS CLEAR: JESUS'S MINISTRY IS NOT MERELY A HEALING ONE, BUT HIS NAME COULD EASILY BE JESUS CHRIST THE HEALER!

The stories we have shared often relate to physical healing, and, more often than not, we connect miracles to miraculous instant healing. Yet the stance of faith is to accept *any miracle Jesus wants to give.*

Why do we make this point in a book about *healing prayer?* We do so because we don't want anyone to end up bitter, cynical, or lacking faith because they prayed for the healing of loved ones who instead passed away. The healing of Jesus is not always instantaneous. Beyond this, there are other miracles in the Christian life as well.

One of my (Maxie's) predecessors as president of Asbury Theological Seminary was Dr. J. C. McPheeters, who lived to be ninety-four. He learned to water ski at age seventy-five and skied for twenty miles on his eightieth birthday. He was one of those beautiful persons who come into the world like a breath of fresh air. The second president of Asbury Seminary, he was a great evangelist, an effective preacher, and a marvelous teacher. He was a person of prayer who exercised a ministry of healing for over fifty years. I have felt it an honor to be one of his successors.

FIVE MIRACLES OF HEALING

One of the most outstanding lessons Dr. McPheeters taught us during his many years of public ministry was about healing prayer. He said that from the Scriptures and from his own personal experience, he had learned that there are at least five miracles of healing that the Lord wants to give us.

1. THE MIRACLE OF THE INSTANT CURE

We have witnessed throughout this book that the power of faith, the leading of the Spirit, and the means of prayer have brought about instant healing. These have been proven medically and scientifically, and we yearn for more of these instances.

There are some who are granted frequent *gifts of healing.* Francis MacNutt and his wife Judith regularly saw medically verified, miraculous healings and deliverances from unclean powers.[34] The founders of our two movements—John Wesley, the founder of Methodism, and Albert Simpson, the founder of the Christian and Missionary Alliance—saw regular manifestations of divine power in the birthing of their ministries. Simpson himself was healed of a failing heart and a lung condition.

---

34. See Francis MacNutt, *Healing* (Notre Dame: Ava Maria Press, 1974).

I (David) was in a revival in Uganda in which there were thirty astonishing and medically impossible healings in a single day, and fifty over a four-day period.[35] When the Ugandan bishop came to my church, not only was my wife healed beyond medical intervention, but there were six more healings in three days—all seven of which were medically impossible. During that astonishing visit by the bishop of a war-torn country, everyone who experienced a remarkable healing was a known leader in the congregation—underlining that this was verified, substantiated, and beyond criticism. There have been three miraculous healings in my family alone, two of them instantaneous and one taking place over a month's time.

Yet this testimony is not as common as we would desire.[36]

Still, we are in an era in which these kinds of manifestations of God's power are becoming more frequent. Dr. Craig Keener has written two books on miracles in our day. Hard data is used to verify the increasing frequency of such things as miraculous healings. One of the more striking discoveries we learn from Keener is that nearly three-fourths of doctors in the United States believe in miraculous healing. He says, "More importantly, over half of the physicians surveyed note that they had *witnessed* what they considered to be miracles."[37]

The era is shifting. We are moving away from a time when we were reluctant to seek healing from God and are now boldly asking God to heal. There is now more openness to believe that *healing prayer is God's idea.*

Our prayer is that this becomes more frequent as more people learn to discover God's healing Presence moving upon them.

2. THE MIRACLE OF GOD'S UNDERTAKING

God undertakes to heal us by natural means.

---

35. That event was a Healing Prayer Crusade cosponsored by the American College of Praying International that was held from August 29 through September 2, 2007, in Arua, Uganda, the birthplace of Idi Amin.

36. The Rev. Canon Alfred W. Price, one of the early leaders of the International Order of St. Luke the Physician, said that in his fifty years of healing ministry, he had witnessed only thirty-seven instant healings.

37. Craig S. Keener, *Miracles Today: The Supernatural Work of God in the Modern World* (Grand Rapids, MI: Baker Academic, 2021), 26.

For example, if we cut our thumb and don't do anything except keep the wound clean, by a miracle of nature, the body heals itself. God undertakes.

He undertakes by ordinary means, through doctors, nurses, and medicine. He undertakes through other people to bring about healing in our life. It's written into the very nature of things, and that's one of God's miracles.

3. THE MIRACLE OF GOD'S PATH TO A REMEDY

God sometimes leads us, and the leading is unmistakable—God was in it, and it becomes clear that God has led us to a cure. Here, medicine and miracle intertwine. Such was the case when I (David) *just happened* to read a medical society newsletter that helped my wife and our unborn son.

Christ may lead us to a doctor, a healing remedy, or a healing community. When it happens, most of us readily confess that God guided in this. King Hezekiah was granted a miracle of nature, but in the end was commanded to use medicine to add fifteen years to his life. (See Isaiah 38.)

In and of itself, God's guidance is a miracle. He can lead us to a source of healing. Sometimes God guides by directing us to a particular doctor, a medication, a pastor, or a friend to whom we can pour out our heart in confession and hear the word of forgiveness.

A HEALING WORD OF FORGIVENESS DRAWS OUT THE POISON OF OUR GUILT, SO OUR CONSCIENCE RECEIVES GOD'S HEALING SALVE.

Sometimes God guides us to the means of grace:

- To a worship service where we hear the Word of God preached and by a miracle of the Spirit, it becomes God's Word for us that day.
- To Holy Communion, where we take holy elements, remember the Presence of our Lord Jesus Christ, and know that God has

performed a miracle, a bringing together of the Presence of His Son, Jesus and us, in order that our lives might be made whole again.

4. THE MIRACLE OF GOD'S SUFFICIENT GRACE

Remember, in holy mystery, not all of us receive the healing we long to obtain. Sometimes we are going to enter a trying circumstance that will stay with us until the resurrection, when we'll enter a new kingdom. It's a common grace, but a miracle in its own right, when God grants us the means to endure through some painful circumstance when we pray in *holy mystery*.

Paul spoke of his *"thorn in the flesh"* (2 Corinthians 12:7).

Much ink has been spilled in debates over what that thorn might have been, and none have reached a clear conclusion. Yet I (Maxie) believe that we don't think enough about the seriousness of Paul's complaint because a thorn is such a little thing. The truth is that the same Greek word we translate as "thorn" can also mean "stake." It wasn't something little that Paul wrestled with day in and day out. It was something that plagued his conscience to the point that he wrestled with God. He prayed fervently that God would deliver him from that *"messenger of Satan"* sent to *"torment"* him (2 Corinthians 12:7).

If you have read the Bible, you know why God did not deliver Paul from this *"thorn."* He told the apostle, *"My grace is sufficient for you, for my power is made perfect in weakness"* (2 Corinthians 12:9 ESV).

The sufficiency of God's grace is a miracle.

5. THE MIRACLE OF A TRIUMPHANT CROSSING

Unless we reach the end of time, we won't get out of this world alive.

In this present age, death is our passage from *life* to *eternal life* if we know the miracle of a triumphant crossing. The ultimate healing miracle of God comes in the resurrection when *"what is mortal will be swallowed up by life"* (2 Corinthians 5:4).

We do believe that we must commit our hearts and minds to following the Savior, even if we must follow Him into death itself. We trust that we will enter into what He has already accomplished: His resurrection from the dead. The words of the apostle are fitting as they describe our attitude toward this aspect of our faith:

> But the fact is, Christ has been raised from the dead, the first fruits of those who are asleep...For as in Adam all die, so also **in Christ all will be made alive**. But each in his own order: Christ the first fruits, after that those who are Christ's at His coming, then comes the end, when He hands over the kingdom to our God and Father, when He has abolished all rule and all authority and power. For He must reign until He has put all His enemies under His feet. The last enemy that will be abolished is death. (1 Corinthians 15:20, 22–26)

It is important to remember this as our hope, for us to live and believe as those who taste life and death and life again. That "last enemy" is still around, causing us to mourn and grieve. Yet death itself is mortal. Death will die, the grave will be destroyed, and we will reign with Jesus in unending life.

A FINAL WORD

The stance of classic Christian faith is to receive any miracle God wants to give:

- The miracle of the instant cure
- The miracle of God's undertaking
- The miracle of God's path to a remedy
- The miracle of God's sufficient grace
- The miracle of a triumphant crossing

Remember, *healing prayer is God's idea*—and He sends us the package of His grace for us to unwrap. Sometimes the present contained within is a joy to discover. Other times, the wrapping comes off, and God commands us to embrace the holy mystery.

Whatever we discover, we should embrace God's invitation to intercede.

REFLECT AND RECORD

1. Dr. J. C. McPheeters denoted five ways that God heals. Does this approach bring understanding to your desire to participate in healing prayer?

   _____

   _____

   _____

2. The scope of the entire book is now before you. What is your biggest takeaway from this book?

   _____

   _____

   _____

A PRAYER FOR GUIDANCE

Heavenly Father, Your Word is very clear: healing prayer is Your idea. Yet holy mystery is also from Your hand. Teach us to walk in humble submission to both. Let healing prayer and holy mystery intertwine. Lead us into the depths of Your love, revealed in Christ our Lord. Amen.

MY PRAYER LIST

Name/Circumstance	Date	Others Praying

Name/Circumstance	Date	Others Praying

ANSWERS TO PRAYER

Name/Circumstance	Date	Others Praying

Name/Circumstance	Date	Others Praying

ABOUT THE AUTHORS

Dr. David Chotka is the founder and director of SpiritEquip Ministries (www.spiritequip.com). He served as the chair of Alliance Pray! Team (APT)—the national prayer equipping team of the Alliance Church in Canada—for more than twenty years. He is an author, conference speaker, director of a renewal society, and a prayer mobilizer.

David has served his Lord as a church planter, a solo pastor, an associate, and as a lead pastor of multi-staff churches in the Canadian provinces of British Columbia, Alberta, and Ontario.

He has led seminars and conferences nationally and internationally, particularly to train people in various spiritual disciplines, including such topics as "How to Hear God's Voice," "Praying into the Meaning of the Lord's Prayer," and most especially "Prayer for Healing."

David lives in southwest Ontario, Canada, with his wife Elizabeth. Together they have two adult children. For fun, he plays the piano and allows his fourteen-pound dog to take him for a walk from time to time.

Dr. Maxie D. Dunnam is author of more than forty books, including the bestseller *The Workbook of Living Prayer*. He was the fifth president of Asbury Theological Seminary. Prior to his tenure there, he was well-known as a compelling minister and evangelist.

Maxie led Christ United Methodist Church in Memphis, Tennessee, where his tenure was marked by a commitment to evangelism, inner-city ministries, housing for the working poor, and outreach to the recovering community.

He and his wife Jerry, an artist, were married in 1957. They have three children and four grandchildren.

A NOTE ON COMMUNICATION

Do you have a testimony of healing that you would like to share with us? We would be delighted to hear from you! Our goal is to encourage the body of Christ through faithful, accurate testimony.

We invite you to share your stories with us.
We are asking God to lead us to medically verified accounts of God's healing power.

You can email us at: hello@spiritequip.com.

Please put "Healing Prayer" in the subject line.

A NOTE ON PROCEEDS

David Chotka's wife Elizabeth was healed from facioscapulohumeral muscular dystrophy or FSHD. For that, we thank God and are forever grateful. In that long season in between praying for healing, giving up, and then receiving the gift of health, both David and Elizabeth were regularly thankful for medical teams, medical infrastructure, and ongoing research, all of which granted us support and interventions as needed.

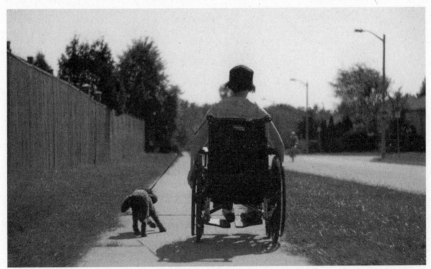

David's daughter, pictured here out taking our little dog out for a walk around the block, has myotonic dystrophy. We are grateful for the medical interventions that have granted her and countless others the gift of life, including Elizabeth's mom, sister, and niece, who continue to endure the effects of FSH muscular dystrophy.

Because of this history, a portion of the profits from this book will be donated to the Muscular Dystrophy Associations in our two countries, Canada and the United States.